CODEPI

———— ❧❧❧❧ ————

No more - The codependent recovery guide to cure wounded souls

Chris S Jennings

publisher or the original author of this work can be in any fashion deemed liable for any hardship or damages that may befall them after undertaking information described herein.

Additionally, the information in the following pages is intended only for informational purposes and should thus be thought of as universal. As befitting its nature, it is presented without assurance regarding its prolonged validity or interim quality. Trademarks that are mentioned are done without written consent and can in no way be considered an endorsement from the trademark holder.

TABLE OF CONTENTS

INTRODUCTION

The term "codependency" describes a pattern of dysfunctional behavior and thought which some estimates indicate affects as many as ninety percent of people in the United States. Like many such disorders, it exists on a spectrum, ranging from mild to severe, and depending on the degree to which it impacts a given individual or individuals in a relationship can lead to more dire consequences than many people may realize. People who are codependent frequently suffer from depression, anxiety, and emotional instability brought on by dealing with perpetual chaos in their lives, and they may subsequently struggle with drug addiction, alcoholism, ulcers, high blood pressure, headaches, and heart disease as a result of the constant stress under which they must operate. In short, the ability of people facing these issues to function effectively, to live fulfilling lives, to realize their full potential, and to simply experience happiness and contentment can become impossible or at least seriously compromised.

The good news is that codependency is not necessarily a lifelong condition - it can be overcome. Understanding and recognizing unhealthy behavior is the vital first step to abate it and avoid the myriad mental and physical health problems that may otherwise be incurred. Once the problem is identified, it is possible to learn new methods of coping, ways to gain self-awareness and change your perspective of yourself, improve your relationships with other people, and allow you to welcome the happiness and contentment we all want but which so often eludes us. If you fear you may be codependent, you can change your life for the better.

The following chapters will discuss what codependency is, what it looks like, and how to identify it. Then, we'll look into ways to break the cycle of codependency and heal to reach a better, healthier, and more fulfilling relationship. By the end of this book, you will be able to put aside codependent behaviors and feel better about yourself and your relationships.

There are plenty of books on this subject on the market, so thanks again for choosing this one! Every effort was made to ensure it is full of as much useful information as possible. Please enjoy!

CHAPTER 1: UNDERSTANDING CODEPENDENCY

> "There are almost as many definitions of codependency as there are experiences that represent it."

> — *Melody Beattie, Author of 'Codependent No More: How to Stop Controlling Others and Start Caring for Yourself'*

What is Codependency?

The concept of codependency first originated to describe patterns of behavior common specifically to people in relationships with alcoholics or drug addicts. These people exhibit a compulsive tendency to over-compensate and make excuses for the behavior of the addicted person, thus enabling the addict to continue in their own irresponsible and unhealthy way of being. The codependent person then becomes "addicted" to helping the other person and to the relationship, depending on it to meet nearly all of his or her emotional and self-esteem needs. It is a static symbiosis in which both partners are trapped and neither partner can change or grow. Though the term has been in use as described since the middle of the 20th century, subsequent research has revealed that the characteristics of codependency are not found solely amongst the spouses and family members of the people suffering addiction but are much more prevalent in the general population than anyone previously considered. It was discovered that if you were raised in a dysfunctional family or had a parent who was chronically mentally or physically ill, you could also be codependent.

In essence, codependency is characterized by a dysfunctional, one-sided relationship. A dysfunctional relationship is one in which the matching of the personalities of both partners results in the opposite of appropriate relationship function. Instead of fostering communication and offering nurture and emotional support, those engaged in a relationship which is dysfunctional - or "toxic" - become diminished, defeated, and self-destructive. A one-sided relationship is one in which partners consistently give to the relationship or the other person more than they receive in return or more than they allow themselves to have. In relationships with codependency - which may exist between parents and children, brothers and sisters, friends, co-workers, spouses or romantic partners - this unhealthy interaction results in a toxic entanglement which is deeply emotionally, psychologically, and potentially physically damaging to all involved.

People in healthy relationships are able to depend on each other. That mutual dependence makes both people feel safe and secure, and that sense of security strengthens the bond between them while allowing them to still maintain their individuality and independence. In a codependent relationship, two people effectively surrender their independence and develop an unhealthy enmeshment that doesn't allow either person to grow. This pattern of thought, feeling, and behavior is a denial of the self and can result in self-loathing, which the codependent relationship partner then acts out through self-destructive or unduly self-sacrificial behavior. Codependents lose themselves in the relationship and in the life of the other person and come to depend entirely on what approval they receive from their partner for their very identity. Their meaning and purpose are derived from striving to fulfill the needs of others at the expense of their own. In co-dependency, relationship partners lose the ability to depend on and give each other support in a way that is mutually beneficial. Instead of forming a bond based on love, trust, and mutual respect, theirs is one based on neediness and unhealthy dependency.

Frequently this type of situation - one in which the codependent person is constantly self-sacrificing in increasingly desperate efforts to attain validation from a partner who may or may not be compliant - leads to a build-up of resentment and anger which serves only to compound the toxicity of the bond between the two and cause further self-loathing and loss of self esteem.

"We rescue people from their responsibilities. We take care of people's responsibilities for them. Later, we get mad at them for what we've done. Then we feel used and sorry for ourselves. That is the pattern, the triangle."

— Melody Beattie, Author of 'Codependent No More: How to Stop Controlling Others and Start Caring for Yourself'

If left unaddressed, the symptoms of codependency tend to worsen over time and become ingrained habits which are more and more difficult to break. Although the narrative may play itself out differently in each relationship, these identifiable symptoms of codependent behavior are shared in common by most, if not all.

Characteristics of Codependency

Low self-esteem

Whether a person's lack of understanding of their self-worth precedes their involvement in a codependent relationship or not, that person will exhibit low self-esteem as part of and due to their involvement in the relationship's dysfunction. Loss of identity and the constant search for external validation keep codependents suspended in a perpetually hollow state where they can't value themselves because they are, to an extent, unaware that there is anything there to value.

Poor boundaries

A boundary is, by definition, a line that marks the limits of an area, or a dividing line between two areas. With regard to interpersonal relationships, a boundary has very much the same meaning: it refers to the implied division between two people defined as separate and distinct individuals. In codependent relationships where otherwise distinct individuals are intertwined or enmeshed with one another emotionally and psychologically, the boundaries which delineate between them become blurred and indistinct. It becomes difficult to distinguish which thoughts and feelings belong to which individual since codependents are so apt to assume responsibility for the feelings of others and conversely to inappropriately hold others accountable for their own emotions.

Dysfunctional ways of communicating

Codependents have great difficulty effectively and authentically communicating their thoughts, feelings, and needs. Due to habitually suppressing or ignoring those thoughts, feelings, and needs, they are frequently unable to identify what they even are. They can be very inaccurate in their perceptions of and reactions to thoughts expressed by other people, and sometimes, they're afraid to be truthful, because of the fear of upsetting someone else.

Difficulty saying "no"

Codependent individuals tend to have trouble saying "no" when asked to take on tasks or responsibilities, even when the assumption of those tasks is a significant inconvenience or hardship. Codependents will feel guilt at the thought of placing their own needs ahead of the wants of others. The compulsive need to help whenever possible, motivated by the 'need to be needed' and to garner approval can dispel all rational thought.

Dependency

One common thread amongst codependents is a fear of rejection or abandonment. They need constant reassurance that they are loved and accepted in order to feel good about themselves. Because of this, many feel that they need to always be in a relationship because they feel too unsettled and unsure of themselves being alone. This trait makes it very hard for them to end a relationship, even when the relationship is unhealthy, and they end up feeling they have no option but to stay and endure it.

Obsessiveness

The inherent fear and anxiety that underlie codependency can cause the people it affects to spend inordinate amounts of time and energy over-thinking. Other people or relationships are usually the focus. They can also become obsessed when they think they've made or might make a "mistake." Other times, they might become preoccupied with fantasies of how they'd like things to be or romanticize the past. Overall, the tendency to obsess is a form of avoidance and denial of what is really wrong in the present.

Fear of intimacy

Many people in codependent relationships are afraid to be too open and close with their partners. Emotional intimacy can be terrifying for someone who depends upon the approval of others to survive because the fear of being judged or rejected and then abandoned is just too great. They may also be afraid of being too close emotionally because they will be smothered by the relationship or the other partner. This leads some codependents to avoid intimacy by becoming "unavailable". This creates discord when, for example, one partner wants to spend more time together than the other partner does. In reality, one partner is denying a need for closeness while the other is denying a need for separateness.

Denial

One of the biggest problems for people living with codependency and the biggest reason they persist in their behavior even though they know something is not quite right is that they don't want to acknowledge that the label "codependent" could apply to them. They will either deny the very existence of any sort of problem or if they are able to admit that there is a problem, they believe that it is caused by someone else or by a particular situation. Codependents also deny their own feelings and needs. They either invalidate their emotions or simply can't identify what they are feeling and are more concerned anyway with what others are feeling. The same is true with regard to their needs. A codependent person will compulsively prioritize the needs of others while neglecting his or her own. Often, the person is unaware or in denial of what their needs even are.

Could you be codependent?

Ask yourself if you feel anxious when you deny someone - anyone you have a relationship with - something they have asked. Consider your reactions when someone disagrees with you or says something about you. Do you react to, or take personally, the thoughts and opinions of everyone regarding you? Think about the last time a friend of yours needed help. Did you feel guilty for not helping, even if they didn't ask? Or did you offer to help, then feel rejected when they said no?

Although you may acknowledge that you possess some of these traits to a degree, it does not necessarily mean that you are codependent. Codependency describes unhealthy **patterns** and extremes of thought and behavior with regard to interpersonal relationships. However, if you recognize that certain traits are leading you to engage in codependent behavior, making it difficult for you to relate to others, you might want to consider the possibility that you could be codependent and begin to take steps to address the issue.

Chapter 2: Types of Codependent Personalities and Behavior

Codependency can take many forms. There are a few different personality models that are indicative of codependency. There are also several types of codependent behavior, with each one highlighting different characteristics.

First, we'll look at four different personalities associated with codependency: the Martyr, the Savior, the Coach, and the Enabler.

The Martyr

A martyr, historically, is someone who is willing to sacrifice themselves for their beliefs. A martyr would be undesirable to government or religious leaders because the death of a martyr would bring attention to the message of the martyr - which was usually the corruption or immoral actions of the said government or religious leaders.

The modern meaning of a martyr is someone who unnecessarily sacrifices their own feelings or needs for someone else. This model personifies the codependent characteristic of extreme caretaking, the inability to say no, dependency, and obsessiveness. The Martyr also has a compulsive need to be "right" all the time and will often manipulate the situation they are in to meet that need. In exhibiting these traits, the martyr feeds the codependent relationship.

The Savior

The Savior codependent will often put themselves in a position where they are expected to (or claim that they "*have to*") fix a situation or person by taking on their problems as their own. They also tend to feel self-righteous because they "help" everyone and never ask for anything in return. The Savior might help the person that is in the adverse situation and take on the results as well-meaning. They take responsibility for what happens *after* they help, even though it is beyond their control.

The codependent savior needs the approval of the person they are helping, as well as anyone who may be affected by their help, and not getting it can generate feelings of inadequacy or depression. Additionally, if the Savior is unable to effectively help the person they are trying to, they may begin to feel unnecessary and either withdraw or act out irrationally.

The Savior personifies the dependency characteristic of co-dependency, along with extreme caretaking.

The Coach

The Coach codependent feels the need to insert themselves into others' lives to offer advice and talk them through the problems they are facing. The Coach will often exhibit controlling behavior, illustrate poor communication, or little regard for boundaries. They don't feel the need to hold back their advice and tend to push their views on others.

If the codependent Coach sees that their advice is not being utilized or listened to, they can easily become irritable and lash out, accusing the person they are trying to help of not being willing to better their situation by not listening or heeding advice born from their own experience. The codependent behavior feeds the Coach's need to feel important.

The Enabler

The Enabler is the codependent model that allows the other person in the relationship to have whatever and act however they like with no consequences. The Enabler will always be the one to "clean up" behind the other person, but not hold them responsible or encourage them to change their behavior, regardless of how unhealthy the behavior may be. They might give money to someone with a drug addiction, make excuses for poor behavior, or simply tolerates the actions of another person.

When an Enabler is engaging in their codependent behavior, they often feel as though they are helpless to change the situation or the person causing the situation. They assume the role of victim, claiming they can't do anything to stop the problem, only negate the effects caused. They either don't understand or deny that their actions are encouraging the unhealthy behavior in the other person, so they don't see how they can change anything.

The Enabler will exhibit low self-esteem, extreme caretaking, the inability to say no, and denial regarding their part in the others' behavior.

Behaviors

The following is an overview of five common types of codependent behavior but is by no means a comprehensive survey of all behaviors associated with codependency. All relationships, like all individuals, are unique and not everyone follows the same pattern. However, in most relationships where codependency is present, all of these behaviors are evident to some degree.

Controlling

"A codependent person is one who has let another person's behavior affect him or her and who is obsessed with controlling that person's behavior."

— Melody Beattie, Author of 'Codependent No More: How to Stop Controlling Others and Start Caring for Yourself'

Control – whether over oneself or others, whether taken or given away – is one of the most significant hallmarks of codependency. Having a sense of control can make codependents feel both safe and empowered but it can limit their ability to live an authentic life when they try to maintain that sense of control by shutting themselves off from their true feelings. It also makes it difficult for them to refrain from violating the boundaries of other people, and next to impossible to successfully navigate interpersonal conflict. Still, people who are codependent don't know how else to operate.

Codependents exhibit a controlling mindset with regard to their consistent prioritization of the needs of other people over their own. They perpetually deny themselves the things they want, and forcibly suppress any unpleasant feelings that arise as a result. In many cases, codependents will develop coping mechanisms involving self-medication (such as alcoholism or drug addiction) or compulsive behaviors (such as workaholism) to avoid or dull the pain that stems from their self-punishment and so they don't have to really feel any frustration, anger, or resentment at their self-neglect. By remaining in control of themselves and their emotions, they are equipped to then exert control over other people and situations.

In the mind of someone who is codependent, it becomes necessary to dictate almost every aspect of every facet of every action or interaction with everybody close to them. They need others to behave the way they want them to behave in order to feel as though everything is literally under control. This means that they have little to no respect for boundaries – either their own or those of others - and can alternate between being overbearing or bossy and inappropriately self-effacing, sometimes, within the same conversation. Both approaches are blatantly manipulative.

Codependent people often struggle to effectively resolve problems between themselves and others due to an inherent lack of assertiveness fostered by their low self-esteem. This, coupled with their inability to constructively express their personal needs and wants, can cause them to choose to either defer and relinquish control when disagreeing with others, thus passively ensuring their needs will be denied, or seize full control of the situation by manipulating others into fulfilling their roles as assigned in the codependent's agenda. It's always a win or lose scenario and never an equitable compromise, meaning that one party or the other is always left feeling resentful, which is not a positive outcome.

Enabling

Enabling is another type of behavior which typically manifests in codependency. It refers specifically to the way in which one person in a relationship will justify or excuse the bad behavior or bad choices of the other person. The classic example of this is when the spouse of an alcoholic overlooks the other partner's alcoholism and actively tries to shield him or her from the consequences of his or her actions. The codependent spouse allows or 'enables' the alcoholic to continue being addicted without having to face any potential repercussions. In codependent relationships, this behavior extends beyond just situations involving addiction or alcoholism to include any situation in which the enabled person is not being held responsible for their weakness, inadequacy, or irresponsibility.

The codependent enabler may believe he or she is helping by sheltering the enabled person from painful reality, but the truth is that by absolving the enabled of accountability for his or her actions, the enabler is sentencing him or her to remain trapped within the dysfunctional behavior pattern with no way out. There can be no change and no growth until the enabled person is forced (or allowed) to confront the truth.

The codependent is acting out of a sincere desire to protect their wayward spouse, friend, parent, or child from harm but does not understand that instead of helping, their actions serve to exacerbate and compound the existing problem. Codependents have a combination of poor boundaries, low self-esteem, and an overwhelming 'need to be needed,' all of which fuel their tendency to want to solve problems for other people regardless of whether or not it is appropriate for them to do so. In addition, they show a seeming inability to disengage from someone they feel compelled to help, regardless of the circumstances. Even when the other person is specifically refusing the help offered, the codependent will persist, reluctant to acknowledge that their help is unwanted because, in their mind, that would constitute rejection. It is for this reason that the codependent cannot see how their enabling behavior does not help the enabled person overcome problems and may, in fact, contribute to making things worse.

People-pleasing

People-pleasing behavior directly relates to the codependent's constant yearning for external validation. Approval and acceptance from others are necessary in order for them to feel secure. They can't easily tolerate anyone being upset or critical of them and to avoid this, they will be willing to do whatever is asked of them in order to win approval and avert judgment.

Codependent people-pleasers feel distressed at the thought of saying "no" to anyone out of fear that they will be perceived negatively. Even if what they are being asked to do will put an undue strain on them, or are objectively unreasonable or impossible, they will feel guilt at even the idea of placing their own needs ahead of those of others. Often, people who fall into this pattern of behavior will overload themselves with activities and overcommit their time. This can lead to resentment which the codependent will not be able to dismiss. Since they cannot reconcile with their guilt over saying "no," they will become trapped into painful compliance. If not, they will worry that they will be regarded as selfish, lazy, uncaring, and a generally undesirable person. The anxiety about receiving this sort of "bad review" and the rejection it implies compels them to go to great lengths to never have to disappoint others by opting not to agree to their requests.

Though on the surface people-pleasing behavior may seem selfless, it really isn't. Like much of typical codependent behavior, it is a means to the desired end – namely, asserting control over people and situations. If the desired outcome is to gain favor and invite praise from other people, what better way to obtain it than to willingly devote all your time and energy to helping advance their personal goals, even at the expense of your own?

Codependent people can be passive people-pleasers too, by refusing to state a preference when asked, reflexively deferring to someone else's opinions even if they oppose your own or settling for less so that others can have more. As with refusing to say "no," the refusal to say "yes" is motivated by the same need for approval and both are employed as tools of emotional manipulation

When this type of behavior enters into interactions between two people in a close relationship, it can lead to misunderstanding, the breakdown of communication, and harboring of resentment. Over time, this will compromise the health of the relationship and of the individual partners themselves.

Self-denigrating

To denigrate is to belittle, dismiss, or devalue. To self-denigrate is then to perpetrate a harshly critical attitude toward oneself. In codependency, self- denigrating can start when the codependent offers help to the other person in the relationship, and the other person rejects their help. The codependent would feel inadept, inadequate, or possibly in the way of the other person. The codependent would repress those feelings around the other person in hopes that their feelings wouldn't be found out and validated. Eventually, the codependent will feel useless in the relationship. This can either lead the codependent to fall into depression or cause them to become even more enmeshed in the relationship to find their approval.

Self-denigration in codependency should not be confused with not being able to accept a compliment or other praise. Most people are modest and find it difficult to acknowledge their successes due to the ingrained habit, but self-denigration is much harsher than simple modesty. Self-denigration is also different from self-deprecation in that denigration doesn't have that humor element, and depreciation is expressing disapproval as opposed to denigration's purpose of criticism and defamation. When a codependent uses self-denigration, they are feeding into their compulsive need for approval and further damaging their already low self- worth.

Overreacting

Codependents tend to overreact to any opinion given about them, regardless of the source or truth behind it. They take everything personally, without consideration of context. Overreaction to stimulus feeds into the obsessive part of the codependent's personality and, in most cases, the low self- esteem as well. A codependent that is overreacting doesn't recognize the boundaries of another person's thoughts or feelings. They just automatically assume that any vague comment is a response to them as a person, making the commenter's problems theirs instead of seeing the commenter as having an issue that is totally unrelated to the codependent.

As is the case in codependent behavior in general, overreacting to a situation or person is a learned behavior. The codependent has seen others in conditions that they believe to be associated with what they are facing and replicate the reactions they've seen or experienced before. The codependent has unconsciously decided that what they are experiencing in the present moment is the same as the last experience, though they may not be related, or the memory is flawed in some way or incomplete (such as in the case of seeing their mother reacting to something regarding their father, when they don't truly know what's happening.) Overreacting is the only way the codependent knows how to respond.

These personality models and behaviors are not exclusive to codependency, nor is this an exhaustive list of what to expect with a codependent individual. There is any number of combinations of behaviors and personalities that a codependent may exhibit. These personalities are built on previous experience and family life. A codependent person can often cover up and make excuses for their behavior and has learned over the course of their lives to pretend and repress their emotions in favor of focusing on others, making it difficult to accurately diagnose codependency from the outside looking in.

CHAPTER 3: TRAUMA, HEALING, AND FORGIVENESS

Like all behaviors, codependency has a beginning point. The codependent has learned (usually from the adults in the caretaking position) how to act and has modeled their behavior after what they have seen. Distressing events contribute to codependent behaviors, be they from abuse or death or any number of events in a person's life. It is possible to move out of the codependent cycle, and this chapter will examine the purpose of self-awareness and self-acceptance as beginning steps to doing just that as well as identify how co-dependency is initiated in individuals.

What causes codependency to develop in the first place?

As stated earlier, codependency was first recognized as a behavior associated with families of addicts- probably because addiction is a dependence on something extrinsic, so it makes sense that *codependent* behavior would be most apparent there. When codependency became widely recognized, families of addicts generally were used to keeping secrets and repressing their needs in order to appear "perfect" to the outsider and from there, developed as a lifetime habit. Codependency began in dysfunctional families by the families not being open about their feelings and needs or allowing their emotional identities to develop. Families of addicts or mentally incapacitated individuals would feel ashamed of their families and welcomed the encouragement to keep their problems hidden away from public scrutiny.

In recent history, codependency has been studied more in-depth. Now, we have a better idea of how it develops, manifests, and heal. It can still begin in dysfunctional families, but now, it is known that codependency can also begin in friendships and romantic relationships as well. Codependency is half of a codependent relationship, and the behaviors have to be learned somehow in order for them to be put into action. A person may be predisposed to codependent behavior or have been through trauma that creates the behaviors. A codependent person may be codependent in one particular relationship, or they can display their behaviors throughout all relationships in their lives.

In general, codependency begins during childhood. It usually occurs when a child has to attend to the household in ways that are beyond their years and capabilities, such as cooking dinner or ensuring that their siblings are ready for school on time, or as a result of some sort of trauma, such as a drug-addicted or mentally ill parent or death of an important family member. Sometimes, a child is looked upon by the adults in their lives as confidantes or is made to fill the narcissistic void in one or both parents. Filling in where the guardians are failing usurps their energy and emotional wellbeing. Thus, their needs begin to fall to the wayside in place of taking care of everyone else. While codependent behaviors may be essential in childhood, carrying the behaviors to adulthood can mean difficult or failing relationships.

Codependency may also have roots in abusive relationships, either child or adult, which is quite traumatic to either age group. If a codependent is in an emotionally abusive relationship, they may force themselves to change who they are in order to keep the peace or live up to the abuser's expectations. The codependent may not protect children in the home from the abuse, believing that they can't do anything to stop it or lessen it, and thereby, becoming complicit without meaning to.

In cases where a codependent is the primary caregiver, codependent behavior can be caused by the forming habit of control, especially if the caregiver role is presented suddenly and without warning. The caregiver is the one to dress, bathe, feed, encourage, transport, and make decisions for their charge. Over time, this control can be hard to let go of since the caregiver no longer sees the boundary lines between where their assistance is needed and the ways that their charge is able to care for themselves. Before the caregiver role is needed, the codependent may not ever exhibit signs of codependent behaviors or personality but may evolve through their new role.

Self-awareness and self-acceptance

The codependent individual may not be aware of their behaviors and tendencies. In order to change the behavior, the codependent must first recognize the signs and symptoms in themselves and then accept that they engage in these behaviors for whatever reasons they see.

Once the codependent begins to recognize their behaviors, they will need to analyze themselves and see which behaviors are to the extreme, and which ones are purely caring behaviors with no undertones of codependency. They have to become self-aware of what they are saying and doing that encourages the unhealthy behavior of their partner, family member, or friend. Self-awareness may not happen all at once. It may happen in stages depending on how close the codependent person pays attention to themselves and their actions. If a codependent person only recognizes one behavior at a time, it could take a while to seek treatment for their tendencies. Adding on to the process of becoming self-aware, some codependents may be in denial of their behavior. They feel that they are not addicted to drugs, or they are responsible (*too* responsible, even) for their loved one's behavior of immaturity or chronic underachievement. These codependents still have not fully achieved self-awareness. A requirement for self-awareness is to listen for negative self-talk and discover how to turn that negative voice off. When you can recognize the negativity your subconscious is creating in your mind, you can then begin to break it down and raise your self-esteem.

After the initial awareness happens, the codependent will then have to work on accepting themselves and their flaws. This may be especially difficult for the Coach or the Savior because these two personality models inherently believe they are only "helping" their loved one and not being codependent. They may not be able to recognize when they are participating in the codependent behavior or could be in denial since the addictive behavior is not their own. However, when a codependent person is ready to break the cycle and stop enabling their partner, recognizing the signs of codependency will become easier. A codependent person may very well need the assistance of a therapist or counselor to help them identify the unhealthy behavior and accept that they have faults to be corrected. For many, accepting personal fault is difficult merely because they don't want to face the fact that they may not have all the answers. Self-acceptance is not easy for anyone facing adverse feelings about their actions. Acceptance isn't about changing the behavior; it is only meant for a codependent to understand their flaws. When a codependent accepts themselves, a path is opened up that was previously closed due to fighting the situation and new feelings begin to emerge- feelings of compassion toward oneself and the ability to soothe the negative feelings that accompany the denial. Often, once a codependent accepts their personalities, they begin to put less weight on others' opinions on them and their obsessive need to please in order to turn the opinions positive.

Both of these are emotionally difficult and draining processes to go through. If not because of the recognition that a codependent is not perfect, then possibly because of the realization that they have to change what are essentially ingrained habits and behaviors. They will face analyzing all of their mannerisms that could be enabling the other person in their relationship and be forced to stay aware of the ways they are contributing to the unhealthy actions of others; acknowledging and accepting one's part in permitting detrimental activities of an addict or other misbehavior is sometimes heartrending. However, accepting the faults and getting past the denial is the first step on the road to recovery.

Paths to Recovery

After the critical steps of self-awareness and self-acceptance, the path to recovering from codependent behaviors and personality opens up and becomes more accessible. A codependent person can begin to see ways to not only break the cycles but begin to heal so they can avoid co-dependency in the future.

The codependent must learn to detach themselves from their loved one in order to be able to begin to heal. They have to learn how to separate the person from the addictive or unhealthy behavior. The codependent also has to learn to let go of the feeling of responsibility for the unhealthy behavior; they can't control their loved one (despite their obsessive desire to do so), and they can't control the outcome of their loved one's decisions. Detachment does not mean abandonment - it is important to remember that, both for the codependent and the addict. Detachment is meant to allow for boundaries to be set and to be able to see the big picture situation instead of taking care to get rid of little mistakes. Detachment offers the codependent the opportunity to step back and view the situation a bit more objectively than they could before. The detachment also means that the partner in the relationship can begin to understand how to make their own decisions and see how those decisions affect their lives from that point on. This way, the partner can gain confidence in themselves and have that knowledge that they are strong enough to overcome their unhealthy behaviors.

The key in any addictive and recovery situation is forgiveness. The codependent has to recognize in themselves their flaws and their function in the continuation of damaging actions in the other person in their relationship. Along with this recognition, the codependent needs to understand how forgiveness works and what it means for themselves and the other person in their relationship. Forgiveness of oneself is most important - the codependent should forgive themselves in order to move forward in overcoming the behavior associated with their codependency to ensure that they can no longer facilitate their loved one's acts in addiction. A codependent also must forgive the addict for taking advantage of them in order to let go of any resentment which will hold them back from being able to move on from their previous behaviors and focus on their futures.

It is important to note here that simply saying that a codependent forgives is not the same as *actually* forgiving the wrongs that have been committed, either from the codependent toward themselves or from the addict. Forgiveness is a process, a series of actions that have to be worked through. Similarly, forgiveness is a difficult process and one that may not happen right away. It's ok for a codependent to acknowledge hurt and anger and take the time they need to process it in order to feel ready to forgive. A codependent should try to understand that the behavior and actions had a purpose and try to find and understand that purpose. With that understanding comes the acknowledgment of the feelings and letting them go with the new determination of setting limits and being kind to oneself.

When a codependent is learning self-awareness, self-acceptance, and forgiveness, they may feel as though the emotions and feelings are insurmountable and that they will be feeling hurt and/or angry for a long time. However, emotions come in waves (scientifically studied, emotions last around 60 seconds) and once the wave has passed, the codependent should be able to decide to let go of the pain. This is not to say that they once again allow the other person in their relationship to continue to behave as they have been, it simply means that the codependent is willing to move forward in a healthier way than they have previously been doing. Instead of continuing to allow the behavior, the codependent can now learn to build and maintain boundaries to encourage self-respect and self-worth. Now, in place of forcing the emotional energy to manage and control or clean up the other person's behavior, the codependent can feel the less draining emotions of peace and serenity, which are needed in order to foster self-respect. Forgiveness will allow the codependent to feel powerful and grow stronger in recovery.

Forgiveness is the trailhead on the path to recovery from co-dependency. Between these three steps, a codependent can begin to heal their past hurts and truly keep their help to actual *help* as opposed to dependency.

CHAPTER 4: BEGINNING TO HEAL

Healing requires awareness, acceptance, and forgiveness as discussed in the previous chapter. For some codependents, they may be able to begin the healing process on their own, but for most, they need guidance from a trained outside source such as a therapist. A therapist can walk the codependent through the work needed to recover and heal.

Once the awareness of the behavior becomes apparent, and the codependent finds their path to healing, their road is just beginning. A commitment to recovery takes work. As is true of any behavior changes, a conscious effort is required and must be consistent in order to stay on track. However, the codependent shouldn't be too hard on themselves if they stumble or have setbacks. The codependent didn't learn the behavior overnight, so unlearning it won't happen overnight, either.

Recognizing Unhealthy Behavior Patterns

Since codependent behaviors first begin in childhood, most therapies involve exploring the relationships from the codependent's childhood and their experiences. Psychoanalysis is often used to examine the behaviors and psychotherapy is the norm for treatment due to the difficult nature in changing ingrained habits and behaviors.

Treatment begins with awareness, as earlier stated. Recognizing the unhealthy behaviors individually is the first step but recognizing the behavior *patterns* may come a bit later, once awareness has been established and practiced. It is crucial to differentiate between codependent behaviors and codependent behavior patterns. Codependent behaviors exist in a wider range than most realize but displaying some codependent behaviors is not always indicative of codependency. Codependent patterns are more suggestive of a codependent personality.

Therapy can help the codependent figure out their patterns, but the codependent has to be the one to stay aware of when they happen and which situations most trigger the behavior patterns. The codependent needs to be willing to go from simply being aware of the behavior patterns to doing something to alter them.

Acknowledging that a codependent has adverse behaviors is where the healing begins. Next, identifying the pattern of behavior lights the pathway. Some people can stay aware of their patterns, but others need some visualization. A therapist may suggest writing or journaling about the patterns and behavior, and there are worksheets available to help keep track of the patterns and keep them in the forefront of one's mind. Writing or using worksheets can help with the next part of healing, which is developing mindfulness.

Developing Mindfulness

Mindfulness goes beyond being aware of your thoughts, actions, and responses. Being mindful includes paying attention to our mannerisms and responses when we interact with the outside stimuli we encounter. This is done without being judgmental of ourselves, just purely noticing in an objective way. Most of the thoughts and self-talk we experience comes from a negative place in the mind. Becoming mindful means that you are able to look at those thoughts without putting yourself down or criticizing yourself. It means that you can see where your negativity comes from. Being mindful isn't focused on "fixing" yourself, only observing yourself.

When a person is learning mindfulness, they will also be learning how to let go of control. A codependent person has an extremely difficult time deferring control to someone else. This is why it is so critical for a codependent to learn mindfulness - it teaches a codependent how to look, observe, and notice what is happening while not forcing their own opinions or actions on the situation. A mindful person can look and see what their good aspects are; a codependent person will have a hard time with this because they don't want to look inside themselves and see what is making them tick. A codependent may see self-reflection as useless or "stupid" because they are afraid of what they may find.

With this in mind, being mindful is achievable in small ways. Think of yourself using compassionate thoughts - *"My obsessive thinking about an incident two days ago is only a habit."; "I stop the thoughts and bring myself back into the present."; "I will eventually have reshaped how I think and feel about situations."* You will see over time that the last statement has come true. It takes patience and practice to reach this new thought pattern, but mindfulness will help attain it. Although you may not believe it in the beginning, these little thoughts will become reflexive instead of the negative thoughts that you are experiencing now. Each new instance of awareness helps feed into the automaticity of the new thoughts. Be mindful of how you are responding to the world and the things that you come across.

Much of the difficulty of seeking treatment for codependency is that the things that form the personality of a codependent are the things that have to be changed about them. They are taking what they are, what they know, and having to reshape it into a healthier version. Not only is behavior modification difficult, but it is also hurtful to learn that everything about you is in some way damaged or damaging to others. When considering codependency treatment from this perspective, it's easy to see why recovery is a difficult process.

Even if you are just starting out on your recovery, you are able to change your thought patterns and your personality. Remember that your behavior didn't develop overnight, so it won't be changed overnight either. A codependent is only now learning how to use the compassion muscle, and until the muscle is strengthened, it can't become reflexive. Mindfulness is not about being critical of yourself or trying to change the behavior - this is important to remember! - but only for observation.

Inevitably, there will be tests to the codependent's recovery. In that situation, the codependent should take a step back, take a deep breath, and allow the reflex emotions to cool so that awareness can take its place. This gives the codependent the opportunity to practice their mindfulness. Taking this one second to breathe stops the unconscious reactions and engages mindfulness and giving yourself the choice on how you react or respond.

Thich Nhat Hanh suggests that conscious breathing helps with staying in the moment when feelings and emotions become overwhelming. Taking conscious breaths makes the codependent pause and think before giving in to their instinctual behavior. It also has the added benefit of putting your body into a peaceful state as opposed to the panic state that the body feels naturally when you're breathing shallow and quick.

Using conscious breathing techniques also take practice, but employing the techniques is beneficial in achieving mindfulness. People generally breathe in from their chests, not their abdomens. Begin your breathing practice by placing your hand around your belly button and inhale through your nose, feeling your abdomen expand. Then, once the belly and torso are expanded, exhale and contract all the muscles until there is little or no breath left. This will help calm panic, gain perspective, pause the instinctual behaviors, and provide grounding if you're feeling over anxious.

The codependent person tries to control everything around them in the hopes of gaining approval from the people who matter to them. However, in becoming mindful, the codependent is making it possible to practice letting go; using phrases like "That's not my job to fix," or "I'm sure your decision will be a good one," encourages them to give control of the situation to the person who *should* be in charge - the person who is creating the problem with their behavior. The codependent cannot take responsibility for the actions of others, as has been stated earlier.

The codependent may find themselves angry with the other person in the relationship due to repeated, intentional adverse behavior. In this case, mindfulness can be helpful in catching the reflexive reaction of yelling or crying. Using mindfulness here may be as simple as a physical release such as exercise or breathing techniques to overcome the wave of anger.

A symptom of codependency is depression, which is another form of anger. Except, depression is anger turned on oneself. Mindfulness in dealing with depression can help keep the codependent out of the downward spiral of depression. Writing and reading about depression encourages mindfulness with regard to the signs of depression. The codependent can use mindfulness to keep from falling into the trap of obsessive thinking and denial in the form of substance abuse or working non-stop.

A codependent person also suffers considerable guilt for reasons that are sometimes either unknown or unfounded. Being mindful of when that guilt begins and the trigger for it can help assuage the guilt or point out the irrationality of it. The codependent can ask if they would want anyone of their friends or family to feel as guilty as they do all the time, or think about the cause of the guilt - is it legitimately something that is a result of the codependent's actions, or is the codependent taking on the guilt from someone else? The codependent will also need to practice saying "no" when the other person in the relationship makes demands on them, and not feel guilty about it. One key lesson to learn in a codependent's recover is that they are not responsible for the happiness or productivity of anyone besides themselves - not to mention, the codependent needs to draw boundaries for the other person in the relationship to begin to take care of themselves. Mindfulness is not just for the codependent, but also for the other person to learn as well.

Mindfulness is another step on the path of recovery. Mindfulness opens the heart and mind to accept oneself as they are and leads them to learn to love themselves.

Learning to Love Yourself

Codependency often results from the codependent not receiving the love and attention needed for proper emotional growth. Along with not receiving the love they need, the codependent has no reference for what it looks like when someone loves themselves. Thus, they can't love themselves in the way they need in order to avoid the codependent behaviors that seek out approval.

When a codependent seeks treatment, the therapist works to try and get the codependent to learn what healthy love looks like and how to turn it inward. This, like mindfulness, takes practice to gain automaticity of positive feelings over the negative feelings that are inherently associated with codependency.

Loving oneself starts with being able to appreciate silence and alone time. So often, the codependent avoids being alone with themselves for fear of negative thoughts creeping up. Once the codependent doesn't have to spend energy on filling silence or learns to say no, they can begin to appreciate themselves because they are no longer focused on everything around them. They are now focused on their own thoughts and feelings. Alone time coupled with mindfulness tends to lead to a stronger sense of self and a stronger ability to alter codependent behaviors.

Additionally, learning to love oneself and be okay alone makes way for the codependent learning to ask for help when needed, and do so without lingering feelings of guilt or distress over not being able to control their environment. Many codependents don't feel as though they deserve help or don't want to be a burden. Unfortunately, many codependents don't consider that their friends being able to help them may allow friends to feel valued and closer to the codependent. Moreover, asking for help meeting the things that a codependent can't do on their own, for example, intimacy can circumvent feelings of resentment in the future when another person doesn't meet the needs of the codependent; the codependent expects the other person in the relationship to just *know* what they need without voicing it.

Loving oneself means taking care of oneself. Many times, codependents are so focused on the other person in the relationship or the other people around them in general that they don't realize that they need something themselves. Physical needs and emotional needs are just as important to meet for the codependent as it is for the people they usually take care of.

Needs manifest in different ways. Relaxation is necessary, and having fun pursuing hobbies or pleasurable activities fulfills a need beyond the basic survival needs. Laughter eases stress and creates endorphins which foster positive feelings and self-love. Pleasure also helps to boost energy.

Loving yourself also means protecting yourself from abuse - both physical and emotional. You wouldn't want another loved one being on the receiving end of abuse, so allowing yourself to be in that position is just as bad. You can't love yourself if you're not standing up for yourself or letting someone you care about tear down your soul.

Another part of being mindful and learning to love yourself is being kind to yourself. Change the tone of your inner voice to be gentler with yourself. Teach your inner voice to be encouraging and praising.

The path to healing from codependency is just that - a path. It is full of twists and turns, beginning with self-awareness and recognizing unhealthy behavior patterns. In order to stay on that path, a codependent should be mindful of their reactions and responses to outside stimuli and learn to love themselves. These things at the beginning of the path will lay the foundation to true healing.

Accepting Your Partner

In a codependent relationship, the codependent was attracted to their partner because there was something about them that they could "fix." The codependent is attracted to people who are emotionally unstable or are not fully in control of their lives. The codependent looks for those relationships so they can fulfill the need from their childhood for feeling needed and having someone to center their life around. A codependent in a healthy relationship will not have their needs met and the relationship will not last.

The codependent will try to take control of the dependent person in the relationship in order to fix what's wrong with them. Unfortunately, the codependent in the relationship will be taking on all the responsibility of the dependent's actions and will quickly become stressed and burned out with the dependent. Even though the codependent may realistically understand that they cannot fix the dependent, they nevertheless try and force the dependent to change. Despite technically knowing that the dependent will not change until they are ready, the codependent still believes and pushes that the dependent will change if they love the codependent enough and recognize how their behavior is affecting the codependent.

The dependent may go along with the codependent's rules for a while, but ultimately, will fall back into their old patterns. The codependent will continue the pattern of control and responsibility while continuing to wish the dependent would change.

Once the codependent decides to change their behavior for a healthy pattern, they will have to learn to accept the dependent as they are until the dependent decides they are ready for change - *if* it ever happens. Learning mindfulness is a good start on this path, along with setting boundaries and learning to let go of the control the codependent so seeks in relationships. The codependent has a long road ahead of them for accepting themselves and changing their behavior; learning to accept their partner will be no less daunting. However, there is a method suggested by Joshua Millburn and Ryan Nicodemus called the TARA method - a four-step process of accepting others as they are without judgment. The TARA method states that acceptance of others is made easier when the codependent follows these four principles:

Tolerate the other's quirks. The codependent might find the behaviors that are characteristic of the dependent somewhat annoying or off-putting, but they are part of what makes up the dependent. However, the codependent entered the relationship knowing that there are some things about the other person that make them unique. They need to learn to tolerate these things in order to move forward with acceptance.

Accept that these things will always exist. If the codependent is choosing to accept the dependent, they choose to accept the whole person, not only some parts. After all, the codependent is learning that they can't change the dependent, so they will simply have to learn to accept the behaviors.

Respect the dependent's need for these quirks. For example, if the dependent needs to alphabetize their DVD collection, the codependent will have to respect that need and allow them to do it.

Note: this principle does not apply if the dependent is a drug abuser. In these cases, the codependent should seek professional help in managing the codependent's feelings about the dependent's need for the dependent's drug use so as not to encourage drug use.

Appreciate that the dependent is unique, with unique needs and characteristics. Turn the negative annoyance about the dependent's quirk into a positive thought. This requires conscious effort at first but retraining the brain to appreciate the things that make the dependent different will allow the codependent to move past the annoying behavior instead of focusing on it. As long as the dependent is in the codependent's life, the dependent's quirks will be, too.

Accepting the dependent as they are will go a long way in healing the relationship. It makes way for establishing trust and a non-judgmental relationship, which is needed for both partners to feel emotionally healthy. It is another way to encourage the codependent to let go of some of the control they thrive on and find other ways to have their needs met or get practice refocusing that energy toward something else in the codependent's life.

If you're enjoying this book, I would appreciate it if you went to the place of purchase and left a short positive review. Thank you

Chapter 5: Changing Codependent Relationships

Chapter 4 looked at changing the pattern of codependent behavior. When change happens, it has to start with one person, the person who wants the change. Trying to change someone without changing oneself is ineffective and unlikely.

The codependent has begun to change themselves. Normally, this results from the codependent having hit rock bottom, the point in their lives or relationships which they feel they can no longer function the way they have been up to that point. Now that the codependent has started working on themselves, they must start working on the relationships that have them feeling as though they are at rock bottom.

Changing the codependent relationship requires patience and time, just as changing the codependent behavior patterns. Changing the relationship takes both people in the relationship in making a commitment to healing in order to keep the other person in their lives.

Relationship changes first begin with communication. The people in the relationship must learn to talk to one another and respond in healthy and sympathetic ways. But communication isn't just talking to one another; it requires listening and reading body language as well.

Developing Empathic Communication

When the term "empathic" is used, one thinks of feeling what others are feeling. This is also the case with codependent relationships. In healing a codependent relationship, both partners have to be willing to step into the shoes of the other person, to feel what they are feeling. Empathic communication means that the codependent is not only actively listening to the other person, but also is to understand how they feel and responding in a way they would want someone to respond to them if they were feeling the same.

Developing empathic communication involves three stages: sensing, processing, and responding. Each stage is the building block for the next, so you can't respond empathically without having first sensed what the other is feeling.

The first stage is sensing what the other person is feeling. This is not only listening to what they are saying, but also listening to what they are *not* saying, both with words and body language. *Sensing* implies that the listener is using cues like body language, the tone of voice, and facial expression to read the speaker's intent. The first step in empathic listening, this is the part of the process which allows the listener to interpret what the speaker is saying and is the beginning point in building the necessary skills to make empathic listening a frequently used skill. The listener has to be sensitive to what the other person is saying, understand how they feel, and pay attention to what the other person is implying as well as what they are saying.

The second stage of empathic listening is processing. In this stage, the listener is processing what the speaker is saying along with their other nonverbal cues to create the whole picture of the speaker's message. The listener demonstrates that the speaker's message is sticking with them by repeating the main points and confirming that they will remember what the speaker is saying.

The third and final stage of empathic listening is responding to the speaker. The listener has to prove to the speaker that they were listening and that they understood what the speaker was trying to impart. In this stage, if the listener doesn't understand nor needs clarification, they ask questions and summarize what the speaker said to ensure they completely comprehend the speaker's message. The responding stage includes using body language and eye contact to show the speaker that you are absorbing their message.

Empathic listening in a codependent relationship is essential to healing the relationship and making it a healthy one. The codependent person needs to feel heard in their needs and the dependent person needs to be able to express their needs, so they don't feel that they have to turn to the unhealthy behaviors in order to avoid feeling whatever is fueling their need for the behavior in the first place.

When a codependent relationship is in recovery, empathic listening assures both partners that they are heard and understood. Healing one's feelings helps to prevent future behavior patterns that are unhealthy and codependent in nature. Empathic listening is not always meant to "fix" the problems that the speaker is voicing; sometimes, simply listening and understanding is healing in itself. Empathic listening listens with the full body - body, mind, and spirit. Think of how it feels to really know you're being heard. The listener is open and engaged, and the speaker is gaining confidence in their message. Now, imagine how the other partner would feel when they truly know they are being heard. This is healing.

The codependent relationship often is not focused on what the partner truly needs, but instead on what the dependent partner needs and what the codependent partner projects onto the dependent partner. Neither of these situations meets the needs of the relationship. However, when empathic listening is employed, the partners learn to read one another in deeper, more meaningful ways. They can learn just the tiniest nuances of a facial expression to see through the façade of strength the other partner is trying to illustrate, and help their partner reach the point where they are no longer pretending strength but actually *being* strong.

When the partners in a codependent relationship feel that they are not being heard, it adds to the stress of the relationship, straining it further.

Conversely, when empathetic listening becomes more apparent, both partners feel more satisfaction in the relationship, and individuals with empathy are better able to manage conflict (mostly because they can put themselves in the shoes of the other person.)

Listening empathically doesn't apply only to listening to both partners in a relationship, but also listening to oneself. If a codependent listens empathically to themselves, they are better able to be mindful of themselves and their feelings. When one is empathic with their own thoughts, they are also more capable of listening empathically to others.

Empathic listening and communication are a solid foundation for a healthy relationship. It promotes healing and respect and builds trust between the people in the relationship.

Nurturing Mutual Respect

It should go without saying that a healthy relationship involves mutual respect between the partners. Unfortunately, mutual respect is frequently discarded in codependent relationships. In order to heal and recover from codependency and a codependent relationship, respect must be reestablished and nurtured. Many in a codependent relationship may not understand how to do this - either the codependent or the dependent. For both, the relationship is built on neediness and seeking the other person out for unhealthy intentions instead of being with a person for their personality.

For the codependent in the relationship, their desire is to control the other person and get them to do as they want them to do - this is not respect. This is manipulation. For the dependent in the relationship, they want the codependent to do something for them but often go about demanding it in a way that is disrespectful and manipulative. Moving past this detrimental element of the relationship requires both partners to learn respect. The interactions between the two people in the relationship generally are not done out of respect but some ulterior motive. Codependent relationships habitually put respect on the backburner as opposed to making respect a priority.

When the people in a codependent relationship begin turning their relationship around, they must understand that respect is mutual and not argue that they will give respect when they get it. This is not the way to a healthy relationship. Even if the codependent partner is the one to initiate the changes, the dependent partner must also be willing to change and offer respect. *Mutual* respect is both given and received between the partners.

Part of giving and receiving respect is setting and sticking to boundaries. Of course, the dependent and the codependent must respect themselves as well as one another, so they are obligated to pay attention to and obey the boundaries set by the other in the relationship as well as the ones set by themselves. After all, if you don't respect your own boundaries, how can you expect anyone else to? If the codependent isn't valuing themselves enough to recognize their own needs, they cannot fully heal and change their behavior patterns. They have to nurture their own self-respect without guilt.

On the same token, a codependent must also treat their partner's boundaries as important as well. Respect is fostered through listening and agreeing to value one another's needs and meet them as best they can.

Establishing Trust

A regular aspect of a codependent relationship is that trust between the partners in a codependent relationship is either non-existent or conditional (i.e., I only trust you if you come straight home from work and don't talk to any female friends.) Codependents and dependents use manipulation in place of trust. They believe that by making the other person do what they want, they won't have to think about how much they doubt the other person's intentions or behaviors. Codependents rarely trust anyone - whether it is trusting them to take care of themselves and make good decisions, or trusting someone not to abandon them. Their personalities simply do not have a place for trust. The dependent in the relationship regularly acts or says things that inspire distrust instead of belief in their abilities. Therefore, the codependent is validated in their belief in the need to take control over the relationship and continue their codependent behavior.

Part of being on the path to recovery from codependency is learning to let go of the obsessive need to control others and establish trust in them. While some people (dependents) need help along the way of becoming a healthier individual, most people are capable of taking care of themselves and handling their consequences. For the codependent, allowing the dependent to take on own responsibilities is extremely difficult. They often tell themselves, "Well, they haven't been able to _____ before, so they won't be able to now," or "They don't know how to ____ the right way." The codependent doesn't trust the dependent to learn from their mistakes or be able to figure out how to properly handle adult situations.

In order for the dependent to heal, they should learn how to take responsibilities for their own actions and behaviors. Otherwise, they will never understand how their behavior affects others and impacts their own lives. The codependent frequently doesn't understand this. They feel that the dependent won't be responsible, so they assume the consequences.

Codependents can hold the dependent back from healing, just as the dependent can hold back the codependent without learning trust. This is why it is so imperative for both people in the relationship to commit to changing behavior patterns and to stay on the path to recovery.

Establishing trust in one another supports the recovery process. The codependent trusts the dependent to handle their consequences, and the dependent trusts that the codependent will allow them the room to take responsibility on their own. As with any other process, establishing trust takes work, time, and patience. The dependent and codependent can't give up and let recovery fall by the wayside if they experience a setback in establishing trust.

With a strong bond of trust from the codependent, the dependent can learn personal behavior management. When the dependent sees evidence of the codependent's trust and faith in them, healing begins to move at a faster rate. As the codependent delegates more and more responsibility to the dependent, the dependent's confidence in themselves and their abilities grow. Even if the dependent experiences setbacks, having that confidence in themselves can help them move past the obstacle or mistake quickly and strengthen their resolve to return to the path of recovery as opposed to giving up. The codependent's trust is critical here.

Actually, setbacks and mistakes can further solidify trust. For example, if the dependent is a substance abuser and relapses, the codependent can take this as an opportunity to show their respect, love, and faith in the dependent by not falling back into their old behavior patterns and allowing the dependent to take responsibility for their actions while still being supportive. The codependent stays on the path to healing and the dependent can trust more deeply that the codependent will be there to help them instead of judging or controlling them. This will give the dependent (often overlooked) the assurance that the codependent will not abandon them for a mistake. This is not to say that the codependent should continue to allow setbacks to happen without consequence; the codependent needs to gauge the dependent's commitment to recovery. If the dependent backslides often and doesn't try and change their behavior, the codependent needs to assess the relationship and the likelihood that the dependent is actually trying to get out of their cycle of unhealthy behavior. As much as it may hurt, if the dependent is regularly holding the codependent back from healing, the two may find it better to part ways.

Once trust is established and solid, the codependent behaviors are further dissolved. Changing the codependent relationship has begun on a solid foundation of respect, communication, and trust.

CHAPTER 6: BREAKING THE CYCLE OF CODEPENDENCY

Codependency is a cycle. In order to heal, the codependent and the dependent have to decide to break the cycle together. Both partners should work together to move forward. For the codependent that is not in a relationship or their dependent is unwilling to change or denies there is a problem, they can still move beyond the codependent behavior patterns as well.

The steps discussed so far that are required to break the cycle of codependency include being aware of and accepting the unhealthy codependent behaviors, staying mindful of yourself, your partner, and the relationship, setting boundaries, and accepting your partner. These are all hallmarks of healthy relationships.

Learning to put the codependent's needs first is a necessary step in the direction of breaking the cycle. The codependent is discovering healthy ways to fill the spaces a codependent relationship previously held, and they are also examining the root of the codependent behavior to work through the feelings their childhood left them with. As the codependent learns the reasons behind their unhealthy codependent needs, they will learn how to fill those needs in ways that leave them feeling whole instead of stressed and used.

In this chapter, healthy relationships and mindful relationship dynamics are examined. The dependent and codependent can see how their relationships can transform from unhealthy, codependence to a healthy, balanced relationship.

What does a healthy relationship look like?

It is a well-known fact that a codependent relationship is not a healthy one. Unfortunately, many dependent and codependent people have not ever had a good model of a healthy relationship. Codependent behavior is learned through observation and experience, so it stands to reason that a codependent has watched another codependent relationship as opposed to the healthy ones.

A codependent person is more focused on becoming the caretaker of their dependent than trying to observe healthy relationships, and then they fall into the cycle of cleaning up and handling their dependents' responsibility and decide that they don't have the energy to look around them. The codependent partner is not focusing on trying to make the relationship work because all of their energy is being used toward controlling the dependent and the relationship or trying to cover up for the dependent.

A healthy relationship consists of two people who want their partner to feel happy, are concerned about their well-being, and be physically healthy. Healthy relationships have conflict, a balance between compromising and meeting one another's needs, are able to be apart, and have a level of support and intimacy that is not controlling. Both people in the relationship have a sense of identity and independence, and though their partner is important to them, people in a healthy relationship don't base their entire being on the needs and emotions of each other.

A social life separate from the relationship is also a sign of a healthy relationship. The dependent and the codependent don't have to always be with one another, and in fact, time apart can strengthen the bond in the relationship. The codependent can become involved in things they are interested in or passionate about, and the time they previously spent in the relationship trying to change the dependent and manage the relationship can be spent in the new activities.

Relationships that are based on mutual respect are successful. Both people in the relationship have set boundaries and the other respects them. Neither partner feels as though they are responsible for the bulk of making the relationship work. One partner doesn't have to cover up or clean up for the other's behavior. Both partners take responsibility for working together to have a successful relationship.

Recovering from codependency requires a change from previous behaviors. Since many people, especially dependent people, won't recognize or respect the changes, the codependent person has to assert themselves and tell the people around them that they can no longer take advantage of them, and then they have to stick to that assertion when the dependents inevitably test the codependent's boundaries. Healthy relationships withstand those tests, even if they are difficult.

A person in a healthy relationship does not control their partner. A healthy relationship has partners who make suggestions for one another, but they don't force their partner to do what they want. Again, the person in a healthy relationship supports their partner.

Once the codependent person recognizes a healthy relationship, they begin to attract emotionally healthy people.

Maintaining a Mindful Relationship Dynamic

The codependent relationship has not used the principle of mindfulness. The codependent person may have developed a mindful practice but applying it to the relationship may not have occurred yet. Healthy relationships use mindfulness in interactions with one another. An emotionally healthy person is able to understand how to deal with conflict and is secure enough to know that they will not be abandoned during a conflict.

When mindfulness is used in relationships, it decreases stress on the relationship and encourages support and trust in one another. Learning mindfulness in a relationship means that both partners are conscious of their partner's needs. Mindfulness enables both partners to read one another's facial expressions and see what their partner is not saying aloud. Codependent people expect their partners to just *know* what they need without voicing it, but emotionally healthy partners know that even though their partner can sense some of their needs, they still need to let their partners know if they need something they're not getting.

Once a relationship begins working toward using mindfulness practices, maintaining them also takes work. Practicing mindfulness as an individual sets the groundwork for using it in relationships. Mindfulness opens up the acceptance each partner needs from the other. People in a healthy relationship accept themselves and their partners as they are. Accepting one another allows for conflict to be resolved easier, but it also signifies that the partners will not judge one another for their thoughts, feelings, and opinions. A healthy relationship with mindful partners allows each one to know that they are secure regardless of disagreements.

Keeping mindfulness as part of a healthy relationship keeps the relationship itself from spiraling into negativity.

Knowing When to Walk Away

Some major points in the codependent personality are being controlling, having the obsessive need to be right, having a fear of opening oneself up to vulnerability and being rejected, and frequently assuming responsibility for the dependent's actions. A codependent person relies on the need of the dependent person in order to feel validated. Over time, the codependent person feels trapped and unable to get the dependent person to do things for themselves. The codependent doesn't know when to walk away, say "no", or deny what the dependent wants.

Recovery from codependency teaches the codependent when they should walk away or assert boundaries for the dependent. The codependent must reach a point where they no longer have the capacity to help, but the demands of the dependent keep recurring. This is the point where boundaries must be set.

Unfortunately for the codependent, *they* must be the ones to set boundaries for the dependent. If the codependent doesn't set the boundary, the dependent will not make the association that the boundaries are legitimately something the codependent wishes to use. The codependent is responsible for setting the boundaries as well as enforcing them. If the codependent turns to an outside person, for example, a therapist, to set the boundary, they will never be able to set their own boundaries from then on out.

Only the codependent can decide when they've had enough from the dependent. It is also for this reason that the codependent can't look to someone else to outline the new boundaries for the dependent. The codependent is trying to move *away* from controlling or defeated behavior; asking someone to set boundaries for them has the opposite effect. Inevitably, the codependent will feel uncomfortable setting the boundary and then asserting it, but they must push past those feelings in order to overcome their codependent behavior. In addition to the codependent's expected discomfort, they must also understand that the dependent will be unhappy with the new restrictions. This is okay, enforcing boundaries facilitates trust and codependency recovery, and the certain pushback the codependent will face will also encourage the codependent's mindfulness, confidence, and offer them the opportunity to further their recovery.

Setting boundaries will help the codependent recognize where their "help" is no longer help and becomes more forceful or more enabling to the dependent's unhealthy behavior. The codependent will learn that it is okay to say "no" sometimes without guilt, and they will see that saying no, in fact, pushes the dependent in the direction of independence and their own recovery. The codependent must learn when to walk away from the dependent and the behaviors that initiate problems in the dependent's life. They must learn that they cannot fix everything and expect the dependent to learn from their mistakes or change.

Once the codependent learns where to draw the line, their path to recovery becomes well paved and less daunting.

Living the Life You Want to Live

By this point, the codependent has learned how to recognize, be aware, and accept their unhealthy behaviors. They have learned the importance of mindfulness, forgiveness, and setting boundaries. The path to recovery and healing has become easier with each step and with empathic listening and mutual respect, the codependent is learning how to cultivate a healthy relationship.

Healing in a codependent relationship encourages consistent learning. The more open a codependent is to frequent and steady education about themselves, their situation, and their healthier lives; the more likely they are to maintain an emotionally healthy lifestyle. There is always something new to learn about a healthy life. Permitting stagnation can lead back into codependent behavior patterns in the long run. Continuous reading and exposing themselves to other codependents in recovery encourages a stronger recovery for the codependent.

With these steps taken, the codependent is on their way to living a happier, emotionally healthy life. They are now able to pursue their own, real interests instead of what they think others want them to be interested in. The codependent is no longer codependent, but instead, they are now a more mindful, complete individual who doesn't have to base their entire being off one person or role. They can now feel complete with themselves as they are.

Being codependent isn't only missing out on what a healthy relationship has to offer. It also causes you to miss out on finding your own identity, your own passions. Being codependent causes you to miss out on true intimacy with someone - that feeling that someone in the world understands you, your needs, and accepts what you have to offer without conditions.

Codependency isn't something that necessarily has a permanent cure. Without vigilance and mindfulness, the codependent behaviors can once again appear and develop into patterns. However, that does not mean that you can't live the life you want, with the relationships you want. A recovering codependent is especially perceptive of unhealthy codependent behavior, so they are able to see instances when codependent behavior makes an appearance. When they pick up on codependent behavior, they have an opportunity to correct the behavior, so it won't get out of hand. Keeping the codependent behavior in check ensures that the recovering codependent can keep their healthy, full, and rich life.

Breaking the cycle of codependency leads to a more satisfying existence.

CONCLUSION

Thank you for making it through to the end of *Codependency: No more - The codependent recovery guide to cure wounded souls*. Let's hope it was informative and able to provide you with all of the tools you need to achieve your goals whatever they may be.

The next step is to begin to understand what codependent behaviors you exhibit and put the tips and information in this book into action. You may want to find help from a therapist, or even someone you can talk to that maybe has been in your shoes, with experience in overcoming the codependency you are feeling. Discussion forums, therapy hotlines, and even emailing with a therapist are a good place to start.

Understand that codependence is a life-long recovery process. You will experience setbacks and obstacles, and ultimately, you may find that the relationship you are in is not for you once you are undergoing the healing process. Your healing and recovery are the most important aspects here, and if you can summon the strength to stick with your path to recovery, you will be able to live your best life.

Thank you for reading! If you enjoyed this book, I would appreciate it if you went to the place of purchase and left a short positive review. Thank you

Printed in Great Britain
by Amazon

KEN VALLEDY & EAMONN CAREY

The
Startup
Lexicon

Demystifying the everyday
language of startups

US edition

The Startup Lexicon (US edition)
ISBN 978-1-915483-17-1
eISBN 978-1-915483-18-8

Published in 2023 by Right Book Press

Foreword

At Harvard Business School, where I teach entrepreneurship, we give students an andon cord.

Andon cords are a key element of the Toyota Production System - used by the company for decades to achieve world-class quality at low cost through a just-in-time manufacturing process. Every production line worker at Toyota has ready access to an overhead cord. If they spot a product defect, they pull the cord, pausing the entire production line. Supervisors and quality control engineers immediately swarm over the line, and production doesn't resume until they've identified and corrected the problem.

The andon cord at my school has a similar purpose. It takes the form of the student's laminated name card, planted in a slot in front of them. If the instructor or a classmate refers to a concept or term that a student isn't familiar with, the student can remove their name card from its slot and wave it in the air. This pauses the class discussion and elicits an explanation of the term from the instructor or another student. The premise: the student's lack of understanding must be corrected to ensure everyone is learning from the class discussion.

If you are a first-time founder, you'll probably wish you had an andon cord. You'll be in lots of meetings where you'd like to pause the discussion and have someone explain a term. If you are with a friendly, patient advisor or a teammate, don't be embarrassed: just do this. But you may find yourself in situations where you don't wish to disrupt the conversation or display ignorance. Write down the unfamiliar term, and as soon as you leave the meeting, look it up in this book. Voila: instant understanding!

The book will fill three gaps in your under-standing. First, some terms seem like code in a secret society's initiation ritual – ARR, DAU, TAM, CAC, DTC – but they turn out to be easy to understand once someone deciphers them for you. Second, other terms may be defined differently by even seasoned entrepreneurs and investors. For example, what exactly do we mean by "unit economics"? How about "Minimum Viable Product"? Does a "smoke test" conducted before you have a working prototype – say, a landing page or letter of intent – qualify as an MVP? Finally, some concepts have more than one name. Witness "fume date" and "cash-out-date". Or "tough tech" ventures – also referred to as emerging, frontier, hard, and deep tech ventures.

Ken and Eamonn have done our community a great service by compiling this volume and making sense of the terms that an aspiring entrepreneur will encounter. If you are a first-time entrepreneur,

I encourage you to carry this volume with you until you've mastered its contents. If you are an investor, give a copy to a first-time founder. If you head up a corporate innovation team and you are looking to engage with startups, this would be an invaluable reference book. If you are an educator teaching an introductory entrepreneurship course, assign this book as companion reading. And give your students an andon cord!

Tom Eisenmann
Professor of Business Administration
Harvard Business School

Introduction

The word "startup" has had a profound impact on my career and my life. Back in 2013, I was approaching my thirteenth year at the global brewer Anheuser-Busch InBev, having reached a senior position within the marketing team as the consumer connections director for Western Europe. On the surface, everything was fine. However, I was in permanent autopilot mode. I had the same Sunday evening anxiety as many people in a similar position and was living a corporate Groundhog Day that was destined to end in retirement.

All of this changed on my regular Eurostar journey from Brussels to London one Thursday evening. Looking to kill a bit of time, I picked up the Eurostar magazine and started to read an article about the rapidly emerging startup scene in Shoreditch, east London. This parallel universe fascinated me – it was full of entrepreneurs who were starting to make a name for themselves, chasing a dream and a lifestyle that made me feel old, corporate and staid. My mind started spinning. How did these individuals lead their lives? What did they do and why did they do it? All of a sudden, I'd found a new passion that would break me out of my Groundhog Day for good.

After this pivotal moment, I started to look for ways into the world of startups – attending events, meeting new people and, most importantly, trying to establish how I could contribute and add some value. I was often the only corporate person at these events and discovered a general consensus among startups that it was almost impossible to meet or talk to a corporate person about a commercial partnership. This amazed me because the technology that these people were creating could provide enormous benefits to many corporations and brands. Not long after, I left the corporate world to pursue a mission to join these two parties together. Fast-forward to today, and I'm the cofounder of a company called Progressive, where one of our key services is to help global brands unlock new growth opportunities through connecting them to the global startup ecosystem.

The idea for this book came about after sitting in many meetings with startups where, every now and then, a new word would come into play that took me by surprise and left me trying to keep up, searching Google for an answer later in the day. I realized that if I was going to become a credible member of this community, I'd need to learn a new language. However, as my vocabulary improved, I realized that other participants in these meetings (i.e., corporate clients) might also be trying to mask their lack of understanding. This, compounded by the fact that the vast majority of these new words were pivotal to the stories that startups were selling, resulted in Eamonn and I putting together this lexicon. It isn't designed to provide a detailed definition of every word needed to survive a conversation in the startup world, but more of a starter for 10. We've picked the words that regularly come up in the average discussion with a startup and given top-line definitions that will provide you with enough understanding to be comfortable using them in conversation.

This book won't turn you into an expert, but hopefully it will provide the necessary confidence to enable people like me to join the conversation and appreciate the incredible opportunities that startups and their respective technologies can bring. Enjoy, and if you want to get in touch to discuss any of the words that we've included or might have missed, please feel free to contact me at www.linkedin.com/in/kenvalledy

Ken Valledy, January 2022

I've always loved words. As a kid, I was the one with my nose buried in a book as I walked along the road to school. That continued into later life when I studied journalism; wrote for magazines, papers and websites; and sent absurdly long emails. Alongside reading, my other passion in life was technology. I was given a Sinclair Spectrum computer in the mid-eighties, and that gift from my parents (which I think my dad secretly had his eye on as a plaything) was the start of a lifelong love of coding, computing and more. The Spectrum's incredible 48K of RAM was my catalyst for experimentation on Ataris, Amigas, PCs, 14.4KB dial-up, broadband, websites, social media, mobile and more. My passion for technology has helped me to start companies, meet some of the best friends and colleagues I've ever had, and has given me more opportunities than a six-year-old version of myself could ever have imagined.

The combination of tech and words is a fascinating one. From the simplicity of the BASIC programming language to GPT-3, over the course of my lifetime tech has evolved at an incredible pace, and the language that we use in and around the industry has had to mirror that rapid evolution. One of the great things about the tech and investing world in which I now find myself is the constant opportunity to read interesting things, meet amazing people who are working on world-changing ideas and learn more about the technologies that will shape the next 10 to 20 years and beyond. It all changes so often that I find myself talking to founders about words, acronyms or slang that are commonplace for many but confusing for new founders or folks who are interested in becoming better educated about the industry.

Funnily enough, the first conversation I had with Ken about this book happened the morning after one with a founder who had asked why there wasn't a glossary of terms to help people going through the investment process for the first time. There's plenty of information out there, but it's frequently missing some key words, facts and context. That's what this book aims to deliver.

Hopefully, as you go through your journey as a student, teacher, interested observer, founder, team member or anyone else in the industry, this book will prove to be a valuable reference. Given how quickly the language in this sector evolves, I suspect version two will be with you before too long, so please forgive any omissions, enjoy the definitions and the stories, and feel free to contact me on Twitter @eamonncarey to let me know what you'd like to see more or less of in the next edition.

Eamonn Carey, January 2022

How to use this book

The Startup Lexicon contains over 200 short definitions of terms that are used in the startup, tech and investing worlds – and occasionally beyond. It's designed to give you an inch-deep, mile-wide understanding of some of the words and phrases that are commonplace in those industries. To liven things up a little, we also asked some of our friends to contribute anecdotes, stories and their own thoughts on some of the definitions that we felt needed to be fleshed out in more detail.

As you work your way through the definitions, you

may find words, phrases, acronyms or abbreviations that you haven't come across before. The goal of this book is to help you learn as much as possible about this evolving language, so keep checking through the alphabetical list to cross-reference the terms that are new to you. For example, the definition of VC appears toward the end of the book, but we reference it frequently earlier on. You can be sure that, if we've mentioned a specific term, there will be a definition of it somewhere in the book.

A/B testing

A/B testing (also known as split testing) is an experiment carried out by companies. They show two or more variants of a web page or app that has a specific conversion goal (i.e., getting people to click "download", get started, sign up now or take another action) to users at random. The results of the test are then collated to determine which version has the best outcome or conversion rate. Perhaps one of the most famous examples of this was when Google tested 41 shades of blue to determine the optimal one for their logo.

Accelerator

A program (also known as an accelerator program) that allows startups to join a group or cohort of other companies for a fixed period of time, usually between three and six months, conducted in person or virtually. Most accelerators provide access to capital, educational programming, mentorship and a network of partners, investors and other companies. Y Combinator, Techstars, 500 Startups and OnDeck are among the best-known accelerator programs globally, but there are hundreds of others run by organizations, universities, municipalities and other bodies. Most accelerators take between six and eight percent of the equity in a company in exchange for a $100-$150,000 investment. Companies such as Airbnb, Dropbox, Stripe, Sendgrid, Coinbase and Reddit are all accelerator alumni.

Accredited investor

There are several categories of accredited investor, but the term generally refers to high-net-worth individuals (HNWIs), banks, investment funds and corporate entities permitted to invest in securities that aren't registered with the Securities and Exchange Commission in the United States. Most startup and scaleup businesses meet these criteria. For example, to qualify as an accredited investor in the United States, an individual must have a net worth of at least $1M or an annual salary of $200,000 or above. The rules around accredited investors vary from country to country and in many cases are being reviewed due to the rise of crowdfunding platforms and other tools that allow individuals to invest in these unregistered securities.

Acqui-hiring

When a company decides to acquire another company purely to recruit its employees, rather than to own its products or services. In general, these transactions do not result in a return to the company's investors but instead involve employees receiving equity or options in the acquiring company.

Add-on service

An additional feature, product or service that companies sell alongside their primary product. For example, a B2B company may offer a SaaS product but also have an implementation package or option that customers can purchase for an additional cost. For example, many artificial intelligence (AI) or machine learning (ML) companies sell a product where the primary revenue stream is a SaaS product, but an installation and training package is necessary in order for companies to understand and make the best use of the product.

Adventure capitalist

A subset of the VC industry. An adventure capitalist's investment focus is on either emerging markets or emerging technologies. These investors typically become involved in companies at a very early stage and are hands-on with the companies in which they invest.

Agile

A project management methodology that has its origins in the 2001 Agile Manifesto, which details four values and 12 principles for Agile software development. The methodology breaks up a project into multiple phases. Often used in software development, it allows for iteration and changes in the product spec. It demands an extremely high degree of collaboration between the various stakeholders involved in the process. Agile teams tend to work in two- to four-week sprints, meeting regularly to review the results and iterate according to any updates or requirements.

Ah… Agile: a word that has been so bastardized within some large organizations over the past few years. But what is it and why is it important? In essence, Agile is an iterative approach to project management and software development that helps teams to deliver value to their customers faster and with fewer issues. This promise is driven by a belief that, instead of betting everything on a "big bang" launch (sometimes referred to as waterfall project management, where you only start a new phase when the previous one is complete), an Agile team delivers work in small but consumable increments. Requirements, plans and results are continuously evaluated, which means that teams have a natural mechanism for responding to change without having to wait for a formalized monthly check-in or update.

If something needs to be updated or changed, in principle it can happen faster using an Agile approach rather than a waterfall one.

What I have come to appreciate is that Agile is based on several values:

1. *Individuals and interactions over processes and tools.*
2. *Working software over comprehensive documentation.*
3. *Customer collaboration over contract negotiation.*
4. *Responding to change over following a plan.*

Although Agile is closely linked with software development, its principles can be applied to many projects. When it's adopted by large organizations, it's important that they don't confuse speed with doing the right thing. Yes, it's crucial to move quickly, but no matter how fast you move, it's garbage in, garbage out. Remember that the customer pays your wages, and you need to focus on delivering value for them and being responsive to their ever-evolving needs and desires. Please remember that Agile is just an approach and doesn't guarantee success. You need to ensure the entire organization gets it and is set up to succeed in order for the approach to work.

Mick Doran, *co-founder, Noggin the Brain People (ex-P&G, PepsiCo, Heineken and Sainsbury's Bank)*

Agile software development

See above.

Alpha testing

This is usually the first phase of software testing that businesses will engage in. Alpha testing is conducted to receive feedback, either in house or with a limited subset of friends, family, connections or investors. Companies iterate on their product after the alpha stage before moving onto a beta release, which goes out to a wider pool of users or customers.

Angel Capital Association

The professional association of active accredited investors in North America. In the UK, the equivalent body is the UKBAA (UK Business Angels Association).

Angel investor

A high-net-worth individual who provides financial backing for startups or entrepreneurs, usually in exchange for equity in the company. Angel investors can sometimes be found within an entrepreneur's network of family and friends but are more likely to be successful founders, operators or businesspeople. Groups of angel investors sometimes band together to co-invest in a syndicate.

> *Angel investing is what got me into this whole world. I was fortunate enough to have some success in business, and a huge portion of that can be*

attributed to the knowledge, guidance and expertise of folks who took time to have coffee or a beer with me almost twenty years ago. Every founder stands on the shoulders of others, and having the right people around the table with you is invaluable. Those coffees and beers were foundational moments for me, and fundamental ones in my journey as a founder.

With that in mind, it was incredible to start getting requests for help, support, advice, a shoulder to cry on and more from other founders as my own ventures started to scale. One of the jokes I told founders when I was running accelerator programs is that we teach them about all the mistakes we have made so that they can avoid them, and go and make a bunch of new mistakes before coming back and teaching us how to avoid those. My view was that if I could help one company avoid the myriad detours and wrong turns along the way, then I'd be paying things forward in the right way.

That decision to spend time with younger startups was the start of my angel investing journey. The more time I spent with founders, the more I started thinking about how I could help, how I could get more involved and how I could stay involved beyond an initial conversation. It didn't hurt that they were all substantially smarter than me, with better ideas to boot - so getting behind them made a lot of sense.

My first angel investment came about after a conversation with a founder who was building a new way for people to work - no more centralized offices, but rather a network of spaces where individuals, *teams and whole companies could come together on a full time or ad hoc basis (or a combo thereof) to work. As someone who had struggled with leases, office moves and more – this sounded like manna from heaven. Someone solving an itch I felt myself.*

It grew from there – from backing people who were solving problems that I had faced myself, or ones that I really understood – to starting to work with people who were solving problems that I thought the world deserved to see solved, or ones that would just make people healthier, happier or better off.

Over the last six or seven years of being an angel investor, I've not only been lucky enough to invest in some great companies, I've also had the good fortune to broaden my horizons when it comes to new technologies, new geographies and much more besides. More importantly, I've met some incredible people and made some friends that I am fortunate enough to be able to support on their ventures.

Angel investing is not for everyone. There are no guarantees of returns. Everyone hopes for a 50K ticket into Uber that turns into 200M – I would have taken £500 for 200K frankly. If you only chase those types of opportunities, you'll struggle to find them. What's worked for me is to work with smart, driven, passionate, engaging founders who want to change the world. There's a chance they will, and that energy they project will attract others – and if you're a great angel and a solid support, you'll be the first intro they make.

Eamonn Carey, *general partner, Tera Ventures*

Angel network

Also known as an angel group, this is a collection of angel investors who meet regularly to evaluate and invest in startups. These networks or groups tend to be structured geographically around specific interests or alumni/professional networks. For example, EstBAN is the Estonian Business Angels Network, SpotiAngels is a group of Spotify employees who invest together and Alma Angels is a group focused on investing in female founders.

Annex fund

Also known as a sidecar fund, this is an additional side fund that provides an extra pot of money to supplement fund investments. For example, US startup accelerator YCombinator has an opportunity fund that invests in later rounds for their portfolio companies.

Antidilution provision

These are contract clauses that allow investors the right to protect and maintain their current ownership percentages even if new shares are issued in future investment rounds.

ARR

An acronym for annual recurring revenue. This is a key metric used by companies such as SaaS or subscription businesses that have subscription agreements. Standard formula: ARR = (overall subscription cost per year + recurring revenue from add-ons or upgrades) – revenue lost from cancelations.

Articles of incorporation

A set of formal papers filed with a government body to legally document the creation of a corporation/ limited company.

AUM

An acronym for assets under management. This is a term used in the investment world to indicate the total amount of money or assets under management by entities such as venture capital or hedge funds, wealth management companies or individual portfolio managers.

B2B

Shorthand for business to business. In the startup world, B2B is used to describe companies that are selling their products or services to other businesses. For example, Intercom is a well-known B2B business that sells its platform to other startups, scaleups and large enterprises.

B2B2C

Shorthand for business to business to consumer. Combining the B2B and B2C models, it's a business model where company one (the first B) sells their product or service in partnership with company two (the second B) to an end customer (C). Examples of B2B2C companies or platforms are OpenTable, Resy and other reservation platforms. Restaurants and bars contract with the platform, which provides a way for an end user to make a booking.

B2C

Shorthand for business to consumer (See also: DTC). B2C companies sell their products directly to their customers. Examples of this include popular language learning applications such as Lingvist and Duolingo, as well as physical products such as Kencko, Allbirds, Ohne and others that sell their food, smoothies and menstrual cycle products directly to the consumer.

BAT

An acronym for basic attention token. This is a blockchain-based system built on Ethereum that's used for tracking media consumers' time and attention on websites using the Brave web browser. Its goal is to efficiently distribute advertising funds between advertisers, publishers and readers of online content and advertisements.

Beta testing

The final round of testing before a product is launched to a wider audience. Beta testing will often take between four and eight weeks, although Google's Gmail service was famously in beta for five years. Beta testing is where a larger group of users and customers will test the product and provide feedback ahead of a full public release. The purpose is to help companies make any last-minute changes or updates that are necessary before a more formal launch or push.

Bitcoin

A decentralized virtual currency (comparable to an online version of cash) that can be sent from individual to individual via a peer-to-peer network (P2P), without the involvement of intermediaries. (See also: Blockchain.)

Black swan

A term used to describe a completely unpredictable event. Black swans are by their nature extremely rare but have severe consequences. In his book *The Black Swan: The Impact of the Highly Improbable*, Nicholas Nassim Taleb wrote that the event must be a surprise and have a major impact, but with the benefit of hindsight and data it becomes rationalized. Examples of black swan events are the dissolution of the Soviet Union, the impact and spread of the World Wide Web, and the 2008 global financial crisis.

Blockchain

Unlike traditional databases where information is stored on one hard drive or server, a blockchain distributes information across all the computers (or nodes) on that network. This means that, in theory, the information is decentralized, and therefore more private and secure than in a more centralized model where there's a single point of failure. Perhaps the most famous example is the Bitcoin blockchain, where the blockchain ensures the integrity of that currency by encrypting, validating and permanently recording transactions.

When people speak of blockchain, they speak of Bitcoin and a chain of blocks connected by the solving of mathematical problems – a process that's now known as "mining" in the crypto world. There's nothing wrong with those early descriptions, but there are now many, many different kinds of blockchains: some public, some private and some downright scammy. For public blockchains, the main problem is that every transaction can be seen by everybody.

Imagine owing somebody £100, paying that amount into their personal bank account and being able to see not only that transfer, but also every other transaction they've ever made. That creates serious privacy issues and can lead to situations such as front-running, where bad actors can hijack your trade or transfer by paying a higher premium ("gas fee").

Moreover, blockchains are evolving. Currently, there's an archipelago of blockchain islands that are gradually becoming connected by virtual ferries, bridges and ramps, thus creating a system that improves the efficiency and interoperability of blockchains. This is a million miles from the first version of blockchain but is undoubtedly where blockchain is heading. People keep talking about the metaverse, but I believe the real future is in connected blockchains that enable the metaverse and technologies such as NFTs. Long live blockchain.

Monty Munford, *chief evangelist, Sienna Network*

Book value

This is a measure used by investors and others to determine the value of a company. In essence, it equates to the total value of a company's assets (including any equity value) minus its outstanding liabilities.

Bootstrapping

The process of building a company from scratch with nothing but revenue, personal money or savings. A bootstrapped company doesn't have any funding from outside partners or investors.

This is a word that will come in useful when starting your own business. I've helped thousands of people turn an idea or passion into a way of making a living, and the crux of my advice for the early days is to maximize sales and minimize costs. Indeed, the way I present this to early-stage founders is to beg, borrow and barter when starting out. Need a kitchen space to start your business? Rent one by the hour as opposed to taking on a year-round commitment. Want to host a product launch? Secure free space from someone who would welcome the community you bring into that space and invite brands that want to raise their profile with your audience to cover the catering costs. In the early stages of your business, think about how you can avoid costs by working with an army of supporters and complementary brands that want access to what you have to offer.

Everyone loves a startup, particularly large organizations such as big corporates and universities. Get to know them, as they have access to people, space, funding, clients and mentorship. When you're young in business, this equates to access that money simply can't buy. These organizations want to help you succeed – and they'll enable you to bootstrap your way to growth. As you grow, you'll start paying for space, tech, talented people and activities to motivate and retain those talented people. This all costs. But my advice to any founder, at whatever stage of business, is to keep a sharp eye on the figures and retain a bootstrapping state of mind. It will serve you well.

Emma Jones CBE, *founder, Enterprise Nation*

Bridge round

A funding round that happens in between larger funding rounds. Bridge rounds provide a top-up to help companies achieve the goals, metrics and KPIs (key performance indicators) they need to unlock a larger round of funding. Most bridge rounds are funded by existing investors, but sometimes accommodate new ones.

This is a round that happens when you haven't built sufficient proof points to raise the next proper round. It's usually provided by internal investors and should be considered as their support to you and the company. Looking at this definition, it seems that the company has not fulfilled its goals and hence feels like a negative. In such situations, experienced investors often ask: "Is it a bridge or a pier?" This indicates that the additional runway may still be too short to achieve sufficient milestones to be able to convince investors to invest the next level of money (or any further money). But even if the situation is difficult, the added time allows you to apply entrepreneurial creativity, which can overcome any obstacle. If you have good investors on board, they may even throw you more than one consecutive lifeline. They may have seen that you can eventually deliver good results and built this into their high-conviction approach to investing. It can be highly valuable to have such investors on board, so try to understand the approach and mentality of your investors beforehand and select the right ones. When you carry out due diligence on your potential investors, you should also investigate this bridge financing aspect and their behavior in difficult situations in general.

A bridge round can happen in a positive situation as well – internal investors may be excited about your developments and especially the outlook. They may give you additional money so that you can raise the next round at better terms than you currently could. It's probably best to try to portray all bridge rounds in such light, as it boosts the self-confidence of everyone involved. To be able to do so, the terms of the bridge round should not be onerous.

Andrus Oks, *founding partner, Tera Ventures*

Broker

Someone who acts on behalf of individuals and companies to help them raise capital. They usually work with a network of funds, high-net-worth individuals and others to present deals. Brokers will often take a success fee and also equity in companies they help. They usually work with later-stage scaleup businesses but sometimes work with earlier-stage companies.

Build verification testing

See: Smoke testing.

Burn rate

This is typically expressed in terms of the total amount of money that a company is spending every month, covering all their costs: salaries, offices, overheads and incidentals. Your burn rate is closely related to your runway and cash-out date.

Buyout

A type of merger and acquisition (M&A), this is a transaction where a company (or investor) acquires a controlling interest or 100 percent ownership of another company. Examples of buyout M&A deals include Facebook's acquisitions of WhatsApp and Instagram.

C

CAC

An acronym for customer acquisition cost. This measures how much an organization needs to spend in terms of resources and costs to acquire a new customer. This is a key metric for investors. The relationship between CAC and LTV is critical, as the ratio between the two can have a major impact on a company's ability to achieve scale and profitability. Likewise, CAC can have a major impact on a company's runway and burn rate.

Cap

Short for valuation cap. Typically found in SAFE or convertible notes, a valuation cap allows investors to see their investment convert into equity at a set maximum price. For example, if a company raises capital from investors on a SAFE or convertible note with a cap of £5M, but raises the next round at an £8M valuation, the SAFE/note investor would see their investment convert into equity at the £5M valuation cap.

Capital

A generic term that includes anything that delivers value or benefit to its owner, e.g., equipment, warehouse, intellectual property (IP). Capital can also include cash that is being put to work for productive or investment purposes.

Capital expenditure

Also known as CapEx, these are funds used by a company to purchase, upgrade and maintain physical assets that may include property, plants, buildings, technology or equipment.

Capital under management

See: AUM.

Capitalization table

Also known as cap table, this provides an analysis of a company's percentages of ownership, equity dilution and value of equity at each round of investment by founders, investors and other owners. Cap tables become increasingly important as companies grow, as investors prefer founders and teams to retain sufficient equity ownership to remain incentivized.

Capitalize

A company is able to capitalize by raising capital, usually in exchange for equity or in the form of debt. That capital will then be used to fund the ongoing expenses of the business.

Carried interest

Also known as carry, this is a term used to describe the share of profits that investors receive as compensation in the event of a successful fund or individual investment outcome. Investment funds commonly charge between 0 and 30 percent carry on the profits they make, with 20 percent being the standard. For example, if a fund has £100M AUM and they return £200M to their investors, the carry applies to the profits generated. In this instance the carry would be 20 percent of £100M, which amounts to £20M in carry. This is then split at an agreed rate between the investment team members.

Cash-flow positive

Accountant-speak that means more money is coming in than going out. This is when, after deducting your expenses from your earnings, you still have a positive amount in your bank account. It's also referred to as staying in the black and is especially important when you are self-funded.

Cash-out date

This provides a rough estimate of when a business will run out of cash. It's a metric that's usually expressed as the number of months before the cash runs out. In most cases, this metric is used by companies that are not yet profitable. For example, a company burning £50,000 per month with £500,000 in the bank will have a cash-out date of 10 months. (See also: Runway.)

Churn rate

The annual percentage rate at which customers stop subscribing to a service or employees leave a job.

Churn rate is an important metric for any potential investor or corporate assessing a potential partnership with a startup. This revealing percentage often demonstrates the perceived value of the product or service in the eye of the consumer, and thus is a reliable indicator when trying to determine business value. Plenty of factors can affect churn rate: price, product performance, service level and customer satisfaction, to name just a few. It ultimately gives a good insight into the lifetime value and long-term health of the business.

Churn rates are incredibly important for subscription services. While working at a general insurance company, we looked at a potential partnership with a telematics provider that was offering affordable car insurance for younger adults. Car-based telematics is a type of "black box" technology that continuously monitors your driving performance. If your performance falls within certain measurements, you pay less on your insurance. In effect, you're rewarded for driving sensibly, the bonus being that the insurance is provided on a rolling monthly contract, meaning there's no long-term commitment.

The provider had a great proposition, but unfortunately the technology often gave customers inaccurate driving scores. It failed to meet customer expectations, and the churn rate of customers dropping the insurance was high, at three months. It was a classic example of the churn rate being a strong indicator that it wasn't a suitable partnership to pursue at that time.

Jim Edwards, *digital innovation lead EMEA, Kimberly-Clark*

Clawback

A type of clause that is inserted into some startups' employment agreements to allow the companies to claw back any stock options from the employee if, for example, they leave early, underperform or are a bad leaver (a broad term which covers everything from being fired for causing damage to the company, bringing the company into disrepute or otherwise being removed). In essence, this means that the company can force their employees to forfeit or sell their shares back to the company.

Cohort

A group of people who share something in common (e.g., a startup accelerator cohort of startup companies).

Committed capital

The money an investor agrees to contribute to a venture capital or other investment fund. Typically, VC funds do not require their limited partners to fund their entire commitment up front. Instead, the committed capital is drawn down on a deal-by-deal or pre-agreed time-based basis.

Common stock

A term used to denote shares of ownership in a company. Common stock (shares) is the most common form of share ownership and is the class of shares that the majority of early-stage investors and employees will earn. Common stockholders also have voting rights in the company but are last in line for a return in the event of an exit, with creditors and preferred shareholders receiving the share of any capital returned first.

Community

Community, or ecosystem, as it's sometimes phrased, is used to denote multiple types of group. A community can be location based – people frequently refer to the San Francisco ecosystem or community. It can be sector specific – e.g., the fintech community in London. It can also be used in conjunction with accelerator programs, as well as online/offline groups who support the various stakeholders involved in a community.

> *"If you want to go quickly, go alone. If you want to go far, go together." – African proverb*
>
> *Building a startup in isolation is self-defeating. To succeed, founders need help from a disparate set of resource providers, including insights from customers, capital from investors, talent from labor pools, knowledge from experienced entrepreneurs and connections from mentors, just to name a few. They also need emotional and social support to endure the hard road ahead.*
>
> *That's why startup communities are so valuable. A startup community exists for one purpose: to help entrepreneurs succeed. These networks of deep human relationships are comprised of people who – through their interactions, attitudes, interests, goals, sense of purpose, shared identity, fellowship, collective accountability and stewardship of place – are committed to the positive-sum game of entrepreneurial vibrancy in their community.*
>
> *Not only can a startup community help you build*

your business, but it can also help you live a more balanced and enjoyable life.

Ian Hathaway, *SVP of Capital, Techstars; co-author,* **The Startup Community Way**

Composable

Composability is one of the core concepts of DeFi. Part of the magic of decentralized finance on Ethereum is that the protocols running on top of the network can be used interchangeably with one another, allowing users to put their assets to work in a variety of ways via a smart contract. In other words, they are composable – interchangeable "LEGO-like" building blocks that can be added, erased and reorganized as required

Confidence testing

See: Smoke testing.

Conversion rate

A variable KPI that tracks the conversion of users/customers from one stage in their user journey to a more advanced stage. For example, e-commerce websites track the conversion from site visits to purchase, and consumer mobile apps track conversion from download to registration, registration to engaged user, registration to paying user, and so on.

Convertible note

This is a popular method through which companies can raise capital from investors. It's an investment agreement that's a form of short-term debt which converts into equity in a subsequent funding round. Like most debt, it's subject to interest, but rather than getting money back with interest, that investment converts into a slightly larger equity stake in the company. Convertible notes are usually structured with a valuation cap or a discount, which will have an impact on precisely how much equity the investor will receive at that next round of funding.

A convertible note is usually used at the pre-seed, and sometimes seed stage, rounds of funding. The main distinction from a straight equity investment is that it doesn't initially have a fixed valuation. Instead, it's tied to the valuation of the next round (usually at a discount; there's an interest component as well, which makes these notes attractive to investors). Besides the fact that it makes the negotiation easier (you don't need to agree on a specific valuation, just the discount), it's also a simpler contract, so the transaction cost and legal fees are lower, and the deal can close faster.

Some investors treat convertible notes as a lottery ticket or exploratory investment – it's useful for them to learn about the company ahead of a future round of funding, but it's not yet a firm commitment. This is especially true in the case of so-called "party rounds" when many investors invest using convertible notes and nobody has a controlling interest or dominant position. In some of these cases, it may be that a straight equity structure and proper lead investor position would compel the investor to take the company more seriously.

With these notes, it's advisable to set an upper and lower boundary to the conversion – a valuation cap and a floor. The valuation cap sets an upper limit that reduces the misalignment between the parties, and the valuation floor makes sure that in negative scenarios or at the maturity date of the loan, the dilution would not be too steep. The loan could also either be converted automatically at the maturity date, or investors could ask for repayment – which is a difficult scenario for most early-stage companies.

In case several investors have invested using a note, companies should also think about how to handle the right to convert vs asking for repayment. For instance, if the lead investor has the right to decide and others need to follow, you can avoid some messy scenarios with individual decisions.

Alongside pre-seed and seed rounds, convertible notes are the main instruments used in bridge rounds. This is useful because internal investors usually prefer not to set a new valuation as well as avoid using the previous one, which can cause undesirable dilution and a negative signal for the company. In this scenario, valuation cap and floor are not usually used. This also avoids creating a negative signal to new investors.

Some people prefer the straight equity deal because it's a better alignment of interest between *the founders (and the previous shareholders) and the new investor. Essentially, the investor who has invested in the convertible note has an incentive not to maximize the valuation of the company – if the note converts at a lower valuation, then the investor gets a larger shareholding. If you want your investors to add value, you should try to motivate them to do so as well, and in general you should make sure that all parties are properly aligned.*

Andrus Oks, *founding partner, Tera Ventures*

Convertible preferred stock

A special class of stock issued by a company, which allows the owner the right to convert to a fixed number of common stock shares after a predetermined timespan.

Cottage business

Also known as a lifestyle business, this refers to any business that is created or being run to give the owners and employees sufficient revenue to maintain the lifestyle and scale of business they want, without having to think about raising investment capital to grow and scale in a less profitable way.

Covenant

A clause in an agreement or contract that states that an individual or company will or will not do certain things. A noncompete clause that restricts an employee from working for a competitor for a fixed period of time is an example of a restrictive covenant that's frequently included in employment agreements.

Coworking space

A space where workers from different companies share an office, allowing cost savings and convenience through the use of common facilities such as equipment, utilities and desk clerk services. Examples of coworking providers are WeWork and TOG (The Office Group).

Crowdfunding

The practice of funding a program, project or venture by raising small amounts of money from a large number of people, typically via specialist online platforms such as Kickstarter, Crowdcube and Seedrs.

Cryptography

This is associated with the process of securely converting ordinary plain text into unintelligible text, and vice versa. It involves the storing and transmission of data in a particular form so that only those for whom it's intended are able to read and process it. Cryptography is used to protect data from alteration and theft and to confirm user authentication when required.

Cryptocurrency

A digital or virtual currency secured by cryptography, which makes it almost impossible to hack, counterfeit or double-spend. Bitcoin is considered to be the first cryptocurrency.

CVC

Stands for corporate venture capital. This is the investment of a corporation's funds directly into external startup companies. The main objective of CVC is to gain a competitive advantage and access to new, innovative companies and technologies.

> *One of the most insightful observations I've heard about corporate venture capital, which I quote in my book on corporate startup partnering,* Gorillas Can Dance, *was made by Silicon Valley Bank's Gerald Brady: "A corporation can partner [with a startup]*

without investing, but it can't invest without partnering."
Arguably, even before large corporations established
startup partner programs (e.g., BMW Startup Garage),
they had established venture capital arms (e.g.,
BMW's iVentures). CVC investments are not merely
(or primarily) about financial return; they can also be
strategic considerations such as gaining a window on
new technologies or influence over a key exchange
partner. Brady's observation suggests that it's vital for
the investing corporation to treat its investee startups as
genuine partners if these benefits are to be realized.

Not everyone is convinced about the value of CVC.
Some think that what startups primarily need from
corporations is their custom, not investment (for which
they can turn to traditional VCs) – thus BMW's Startup
Garage was based on the notion of the venture client,
whereby selected startups would have BMW as one of
their first clients. Others say that it's better for a large
corporation to partner with startups (without an equity
investment) or to acquire them outright, should they
be strategically relevant. My own view is that CVC has
a useful role to play in terms of strategic investments in
fairly mature startups – and that nonequity partnering
will continue to be important for relatively earlier-stage
startups. In either case, as Brady pointed out, what's
important is the need for a partnering orientation. And
that's likely to distinguish the wheat from the chaff
when it comes to CVC investors.

Shameen Prashantham, *professor of international
business and strategy, China Europe International
Business School*

DAO

Stands for decentralized autonomous organization. A DAO is a community-led entity that runs online via blockchain, governed entirely by its individual members rather than the traditional central authority of a board of members or executives.

DAPP

Decentralized applications (also known as dApps or dapps) are digital applications that run on a blockchain. Due to their decentralized nature, DAPPs provide many privacy advantages, as users don't need to submit personal information to use the product, relying instead on smart contracts.

DAU

An acronym for daily active users, meaning the number of unique users that interact with a product (e.g., an app) within a one-day window.

Deal flow

A term used by investors and others to describe a flow of investment opportunities. This is usually a combination of inbound/cold emails, deals that emerge from investors' existing networks of friends, portfolio companies and others, as well as any proprietary deal flow they may have through private networks, university relationships and more.

Deal lead

An individual at a VC fund who is the designated champion of the deal. On most occasions this will be the principal or partner, who leads on the communications with the company and acts as their internal advocate within the fund. The deal lead also defines the deal terms such as investment amount, valuation and more.

Deal structure

The terms of an agreement between a company and their investors. For most startups, deals are either priced (or equity) rounds or convertible note rounds, with a smaller number involving a combination of both. The deal structure also includes the rights and responsibilities that the startup and investor undertake.

Debt financing

A type of financing where a company borrows money to manage the business rather than financing through equity (the issuing of shares). Examples of debt financing are bank loans, personal loans and credit cards. In the case of startups, debt financing usually comes from specific venture debt funds and companies as well as from companies such as Clearbanc and Uncapped, which deal in revenue and inventory-based funding.

Decacorn

A company worth in excess of $10B. Decacorn is a portmanteau of "unicorn" (a company with a billion-dollar-plus valuation) and "deca" (meaning 10, from the Greek *deka*).

DeFi

Stands for decentralized finance. DeFi is a blockchain-based form of finance that doesn't rely on central financial intermediaries such as banks and exchanges to offer traditional financial instruments. DeFi leverages smart contracts on blockchains, the most common for this purpose being Ethereum.

Decentralized web

Also known as DWeb, this is similar to the World Wide Web that we know but doesn't rely on centralized operators (Facebook or Google, for example). Individuals will own the content that they post and can control and benefit from it financially.

Demo day

This usually happens at the end of accelerator programs, although there are several online versions that are run separately. Demo day is an online or virtual event where a number of companies that are part of an accelerator cohort or other group have an opportunity to pitch or demo their products and services to an external audience. The primary audience of these demo days are angel investors and VCs, although in many cases a wider group of attendees are involved.

Dilution

When a company raises capital or allocates some shares to an option pool or co-founder, the resulting decrease in the shareholding of other shareholders is referred to as dilution. For example, in a business that raises a $1M pre-seed round at a $5M post-money valuation (i.e., after investment has been made), the existing shareholders will be diluted by 20 percent.

Dilution protection

A clause in a term sheet or investment agreement that protects an investor's stake in the company from dilution in a subsequent round or rounds of investment. (See also: Antidilution provision.)

Disclosure document

A legal document exchanged by founders and investors that discloses any potential issues that could have an impact on the company or investment. For example, if a company is in debt or being sued, they would need to inform an investor in a disclosure document or letter. This is closely related to an NDA.

Disruptors

Many tech companies are (or think of themselves as) disruptors, in that they come into an existing market or segment of the economy and apply technology to speed up processes or make them more efficient. In doing so, they rapidly gain market share and disrupt the incumbents in that space. One of the best examples of this is the way in which Uber and other ride-hailing apps disrupted the more traditional taxi license markets around the world.

DLT

Shorthand for distributed ledger technology. This is a secure digital system for recording the transaction of assets in which the transactions and their respective details are recorded in numerous places at the same time. Unlike traditional databases, distributed ledgers have no central data store or administration functionality. Blockchain is a well-known example of a distributed ledger technology.

Double bottom line

Also known as DBL or 2BL, this is a metric that covers not only the traditional bottom line, such as profitability or growth, but also an additional one that's related to how much of a positive social impact a business is having. One of the best-known examples of this is Ben & Jerry's ice cream, which had both business and social objectives – profit and community impact.

Down round

A round of funding raised by a startup where the valuation is lower than the valuation in the previous round of funding. Many companies (such as Soundcloud, Flipkart, Foursquare and TaskRabbit) have had down rounds. In general, the founders and team, as well as previous investors, suffer substantial dilution in a down round scenario, particularly if there are antidilution clauses in any of the previous investment documents.

In the life of a tech founder, raising a funding round is usually synonymous with success, and tends to indicate growth. So when one hears the words "down round" for the first time, introduced by existing or (worse) potential investors, it's as if an earthquake just shook them at their core! They are dirty words, like black clouds heralding the inevitable doom – the end of the growth trajectory of their company. That same growth is so dearly desired but, if we're being honest, most of the time it's forced upon them by the tech industry and its virtuous/vicious circle of ever-increasing valuations. But if you think about it (and it's oh-so-easy from the outside), a down round can often be a lifeline for an otherwise dying company. So, yes, it's hard to hear, but down rounds are often a blessing in disguise, a much-needed reset, and a way to refocus the strategy and restart the business on a new path towards success.

One such company I invested in and supported along the way got pushed by institutional investors into a very high valuation too quickly without the validation of the market. It was a classic case of "too fast go-to-market" with "not enough of a product/ market fit". This resulted in a battle to the bottom on the next down round as no one was ready to invest so high. Fast-forward a year, and the company is in much better shape than before, with more potential to grow than they ever thought possible. Not so bad after all.

Raph Crouan, *founder and CEO, DisruptVenture Ltd*

Downstream integration

Also known as forward integration, this is a business strategy that's used when a company looks to own or control activities that are down the line in the value chain (i.e., control of its distribution or logistical activities). Perhaps the most well-known example of this is Amazon. They started as a marketplace that held no stock, simply passing the orders on to publishers. Three years later, they made the decision to rent a warehouse and own stock. Fifteen years on, they have their own delivery fleets of aircraft and trucks.

Drive-by deal

This is where an investor puts capital into a company in the hope of a fast return. These deals typically happen at the pre-IPO stage, when a return is all but guaranteed. They generally involve minimal due diligence and participation/support by the VC or investor in question.

DTC

Shorthand for direct to consumer, this is a subset of the B2C market. The term is generally used to refer to companies that sell physical products to customers on a one-off or subscription basis. For the most part, these are brands that are digital-first in that they don't have a physical retail location where customers can try or test the product before they buy. Some well-known examples of DTC brands include the footwear brand Allbirds, the subscription food companies HelloFresh and Kencko, and the mattress company Casper.

Due diligence

A process that investors and others follow in order to dig into the structure of a company. It's generally run by VC and angel investors to look at the accounts, legal agreements and other data that a business holds before deciding to make an investment. As a rule, this happens at the final stages of the investment decision process. Think of it as a background check on you, your company and your business to date. Due diligence (or DD, as many refer to it) is usually light in early-stage investments but becomes increasingly detailed as the size of investment increases.

Early adopters

These are the first users of a product. They're often key influencers who are active on social media and tend to offer you brutally honest and direct feedback. If you can identify these people effectively and interact with them at an early stage, you can expect plenty of free brand exposure through personal endorsements and recommendations.

Early exit

When startup owners sell their ownership before they planned to, rather than when the business is at growth stage. This could often be to liquidate financial assets to safely exit from the market and minimize losses, or to take advantage of earlier-than-expected gains. In other instances, an early exit takes place when a company is building a product or technology that a larger or equivalent company wants to buy as quickly as possible.

Early stage

Companies in this category are usually within their first 12-18 months and are still trying to achieve product/market fit. In many cases, they're trying to raise funding, build an MVP, secure patents, attract initial customers or partnerships, or move from an idea through alpha- and beta-release versions of their product.

Earn-out clause

This is a common feature of merger and acquisition (M&A) deals. An earn-out clause applies when a percentage of the agreed sale price is deferred until a later date, and is released based on specific durations of time or other KPIs being met. These could be financial or growth metrics. Earn-out clauses are generally included to create an incentive for the founders and team members of the company being acquired to remain at the acquiring company for a sufficient period of time to ensure a full and successful handover and transition.

EIS

Stands for Enterprise Investment Scheme. This is a UK government scheme designed to encourage investment in early-stage private companies. Typically used by angels and VCTs, EIS investments entitle the investor to several tax incentives, including the ability to write off 30 percent of the value of the investment against their tax bill, a further tax relief on any losses incurred, exemption from capital gains tax on profits realized, and more. Companies that raise funds using EIS have often previously raised using SEIS.

Elevator pitch

A brief presentation that features a clear idea for a product, service or project. The name originates from the pitch being delivered in the time it takes to ride in an elevator, which is usually about 30 seconds. The objective is to make sure you're ready to share key facts with anyone at any time in an attempt to convince others you have an idea worth investing in.

The elevator pitch is the initial flirtation in the courtship between company and investor. It's the first – but potentially most crucial – step in the fundraising journey.

An effective elevator pitch persuades the investor to take an email. The cover email inspires the investor to open the pitch deck. The pitch deck warrants a meeting. The meeting motivates the arrangement of a second meeting, joined by colleagues. The second meeting leads to a review of the data room materials. The data room materials warrant reference checks and follow-up meetings. References and meetings lead to more intensive due diligence. Due diligence results in a term sheet. The term sheet guides the legal negotiation. The legal negotiation culminates with money in the bank and a new marriage of company and investor. But it all starts with the elevator pitch.

Daniel Glazer, *London managing partner, Wilson Sonsini*

Enterprise

An alternative name for a business or corporation.

Entrepreneur-in-residence

A (usually short-term) position taken on by successful serial entrepreneurs in between startups or ventures, often at a venture capital fund, to understand the VC side, build their network and gain access to new opportunities. The role often includes seeking out and vetting startups, acting as a consultant on portfolio companies and involvement in deals with the investment team.

Equity financing

The procedure by which capital is raised through selling company shares to the public, institutional or financial investors. This differs from convertible note rounds, as the price per share and valuation of the company is clearly defined in advance and makes it clear what dilution founders, team members, existing investors and others will take.

Equity kicker

In some cases where companies are raising venture debt or other forms of later-stage financing, funds can add in a requirement for equity in the company alongside the return of the principal loan amount and any interest incurred. In most cases, this results in a slightly reduced interest rate or other preferential terms.

Escrow

A legal concept whereby an asset or escrow money is held by a third party on behalf of two other parties that are in the process of completing a transaction. These escrow assets/fees will then be released when receiving the appropriate instructions from the respective parties and/or until the fulfillment of predetermined contractual obligations.

ETH

Also known as Ether, ETH is the cryptocurrency of the Ethereum network and is one of the most popular and frequently used cryptocurrencies alongside Bitcoin. Ether was originally started as a cryptocurrency that would be complementary to Bitcoin, but has grown substantially in its own right.

Ethereum blockchain

This is a blockchain platform with its own cryptocurrency called Ether (ETH) or Ethereum, and with its own programming language called Solidity.

Evergreen

A fund that is regularly replenished – either via cash flow or limited partners – rather than one that has to raise capital every three to five years. Many corporate VC funds are evergreen, with their investment capital coming off the balance sheet. Likewise, family offices and ultra-high-net-worth individual funds do not have external limited-partners or investors and so could be classed as evergreen.

Exit

This occurs when a startup or business sells some or all of their company to another business. In the majority of cases, this means the whole company is acquired, including assets and team members. The goal for most investors is an exit that provides the highest possible return on their investment.

Exit strategy

A plan that lays down how a business owner plans to sell their company to give them and their investors the best possible return on their investment. This can be in the form of an IPO, a trade sale, M&A, a fire sale and more.

F

Fire sale

A fire sale is an urgent sale of a company or its assets at a price that is far below its market value. This most often happens when a company is running out of capital and wants to avoid liquidation or receivership.

First-mover advantage

Simply defined as a company's ability to be better off than its competitors as a result of being the first to market in a new product category/sector.

> *"First to market wins." This is the advice of Leonard Lauder in his book* The Company I Keep. *I've seen this myself, and more than nine years after founding SoPost, I'm experiencing the benefits of being first on a daily basis. Because our company was so unique in what we offered, I had a major advantage: the only thing I really needed to do was convince brands that they should be distributing product samples online rather than through more conventional channels. If they agreed with my reasoning, it was pretty much a given that SoPost would be the partner they'd do it with. After all, there weren't really any viable*

alternatives. This meant that we won more business than if we were in a crowded market, or if we were the second, third or fourth company to enter the space. And, of course, everything compounds. Because our success rate was so high, we grew a lot faster than we otherwise would have.

Our advantage endures to this day. We have a reputation as the leading company in our space, and our head start means that we have more data with which to build incredible experiences, more insight into the market and, frankly, the greatest drive to keep innovating. While we're building the future of product sampling, all I see from those following in our footsteps are hasty attempts to catch up. I know who I'd bet on to win.

Jonathan Grubin, *founder and CEO, SoPost*

Flat round

A round of raising finance that is closed at the same valuation as the startup's previous round of financing. In many cases, this happens as part of a bridge round or in cases where a company has been unable to deliver on some KPIs that they promised in their conversations with previous round investors.

Founder burnout

A form of exhaustion caused by constantly feeling overwhelmed when founding and building a business from scratch. Like other forms of burnout, it happens as a direct result of excessive and prolonged emotional, mental and physical stress.

This founder burnout story started at 2 am one day, when an ambulance had to be called because, despite being 36 and healthy, I was experiencing chest pain. At the time, my co-founder and I were running our second startup (we'd had a small exit from the first) and our marketing tech was being used by brands such as Vodafone, Expedia and Samsung. Unbeknown to me at the time, this was the first sign that I had a form of posttraumatic stress caused by the relentless pace and pressure to perform that I put myself under as a founder. By the point of diagnosis 17 months later, I was having completely unprompted panic attacks, even while walking my dog in the park.

This is just one story, but it turns out mine was far from the only one. According to the Entrepreneur Pressure & Wellbeing Report 2019, nine out of ten founders show signs of mental health strain, with 78 percent believing that running their business has affected their mental health and 68 percent experiencing regular sleep issues. If this isn't enough, almost everyone believes they're the only one struggling with challenges as a founder, leaving eight out of ten alone on the entrepreneurial roller coaster. As founders, we all know we need to set ourselves up for a marathon, not a sprint, but these stats stop us going the distance. That's why we created FounderCircles, intimate and safe coaching spaces for founders to problem-solve together, share knowledge and support each other, stopping loneliness in its tracks and creating real connection that fuels founders to be resilient and thrive, not just survive on the journey.

Christina Richardson, *founder, weare3Sixty*

Founder/market fit

A phrase used by some investors to talk about the experience a founder has in the sector in which they're doing business. For example, someone who has been a lawyer for ten years and is now starting a legal tech business to address a problem they faced in their career would be deemed to have strong founder/market fit.

Fungible token

In cryptocurrency terms, a fungible token refers to a uniform token that can be exchanged with other, similar cryptocurrencies. For example, the cryptocurrency Bitcoin is a common example of a digital fungible token, where if you send somebody a bitcoin and they send you one back, it doesn't need to be the same bitcoin. This same concept of fungibility exists with fiat currencies as well. If you give someone a five-pound note, they can repay you with any other five-pound note rather than having to give you back the original one you gave them.

Fume date

The estimated date when a company will run out of money (See also: Cash-out date).

Fund of funds

An investment vehicle that invests in other VC or private equity investment vehicles. The goal of these is to achieve a broad degree of diversification of the types of funds or investments they're making across multiple sectors and asset classes.

Funding round

Used to describe the rounds of funding that startups go through to raise capital, with each round involving the business accepting at least one investment from at least one investor within a specific time period.

Futurecorn

A fast-growing business set to achieve unicorn status and gain a $1B valuation. Most futurecorns are valued between $250M and $1B. They are sometimes known as soonicorns.

Game-Fi

An amalgam of gaming and decentralized finance, which is sometimes referred to as "play to earn". The vast majority of these games are blockchain based and supported by an in-game currency, a marketplace and a unique token economy, which is usually managed and governed by the community itself.

Gas

Every transaction on Ethereum requires gas, which is a small amount of ETH paid to the network. Gas is the fuel that powers Ethereum and is measured in gwei, a small denomination of ETH. So-called gas costs on the Ethereum blockchain have given rise to a variety of competitive cryptocurrencies and blockchains, many with more environmentally and financially sustainable goals.

Ground floor

The term used to describe the very beginning of a venture or startup. Many investors will talk about getting into a company on the ground floor to denote how early they became involved in a company or sector.

Growth hacking

A term first coined by Sean Ellis of Dropbox to describe a marketing technique that focuses on quickly finding scalable growth through nontraditional and inexpensive tactics such as making use of mailing lists, referral programs or social media. Airbnb, Uber, Zynga and others made great use of several of these techniques.

Hockey stick

An expression used by investors to describe the shape of the growth curve they want to see in the businesses in which they invest. They want their startups to be growing quickly and at least doubling sales year-on-year. In some cases, this can be referred to as a J curve.

Incubator

An organization set up to support early-stage startups with the intention of helping them grow their businesses, progress and succeed. For the most part, incubators work with companies at the ideation stage before a product or team has been fully created.

Institutional investors

Entities such as VC funds, hedge funds, mutual funds and others. Typically, they invest capital that is pooled from multiple limited partners or other sources. Historically, institutional investors have been investors in later-stage rounds of a company's growth, but they're increasingly investing in the pre-seed and seed stage.

Investor FAQ

An investor FAQ is a lightweight and easy-to-manage tool to support your prospective investors, existing investors and colleagues to stay informed and help you close your round and get back to growing your business. Investor FAQs can be included in pitch presentations, or hosted online to provide easy access to the frequently asked questions that companies will get as they go through the fundraising process.

> *At SAP.iO Foundry, powered by Techstars Accelerator, we recently organized a series of great investor workshops with a number of leading Berlin VCs and our companies. The format was a private "ask me anything" (AMA) style fireside chat/workshop where our founders could ask the "stupid" questions and get personal tips and advice on how to raise money from industry veterans.*
>
> *We covered several of the expected topics like how to get introductions, the importance of researching your investors and how important it is to prepare your materials in advance (more on this later) but when one investor (the awesome Ricardo Sequerra from Cherry Ventures) talked about the power of a "Dynamic Investor FAQ" document, I was sold.*
>
> *Ricardo told a story of a London-based founder who they felt was a master at fundraising. The founder had very effectively used a live Google Doc as their investor FAQ to help win over more investors and build more momentum in their round.*

Here is how it worked.

Every time the founder met with an investor, they kept track of the new and unexpected questions they had received.

As this was usually a new question, the founder would often forget to include some important detail in their initial answer or else they would think of a much better answer after the meeting when chatting with their other co-founders and mentors

Rather than leaving the investor to just rely on their original answer, the founder would then spend more time on the answer post-meeting and write up a better, more concise and articulate version of the answer, including any relevant data and links to support it.

They would then include this answer in their follow-up email to the investor, saying something like, "Thank you for your time today… really enjoyed it… You asked a great question about X during our meeting and I don't think I did a great job of answering it. Please see the answer I would have liked to have given you. If you or your colleagues have any other questions please let me know or you can see our Investor FAQ document here."

I liked this for four reasons:

1. It helps build a better impression

The founder used this to recover from an unexpected question and have an excuse to follow up and impress the investor with a better answer later. This shows investors that the founder listened to the question and was quick to follow up (a key skill in fundraising and sales). I like seeing this level of thoughtfulness.

2. It helps build momentum
Every time a new question arose, it got added to the FAQ document that had been shared with all other investors they met. So when the founder was sending out their next email update to prospective investors, they could include a section that was called "New Investor Questions" added to our FAQ document with a list of the two or three new questions and a link to the answers in the FAQ. This is a very worthwhile reason to be sending an update… and subtly sends the signal that your round is probably building momentum as you are meeting other investors.

3. It helps your investors sell you internally
Once you move past angel investors, you typically have to convince or interact with an investment firm, which usually consists of other investors and partners that need to be "sold" by your internal champion. This document helps them sell you when you are not in the room.

Obviously, no one knows (or should know) the business as well as the founders, so your FAQs help ensure internal debates are better informed. I've seen firms pull out of deals when they got confused internally on certain core details of a deal and made incorrect assumptions. Yes, this is probably a sign that your internal champion was not prepared enough, but people are busy, and a handy FAQ document they can open during a debate can help sway a deal.

Finally, it helps your existing (aka inside) investors when they are pitching you to other investors. I know I sometimes get the details wrong when talking about my portfolio companies, so a handy FAQ would help me when I get questions from investors that I know when I'm trying to pitch your business.

4. It helps you communicate internally with your team

I know when I was fundraising I did a great job engaging with investors and managing my pipeline. I was focused on the goal and spent weeks away from the office on roadshows to either London, New York or San Francisco.

However, I failed miserably at keeping my team updated on progress and all the new questions and answers I was getting from investors. An investor FAQ document like this would have been a great internal communication tool for my team and new hires. It would have helped them get a real picture of what investors were interested in and how the CEO was answering them. Equally, the team could have helped me answer these questions which would have a) provided better answers to my FAQs and b) helped the team understand and participate more in the funding process.

Connor Murphy, *founder, Bridge*

IPO

Acronym for initial public offering. This is a sale of company stock to the public for the first time on a recognized stock exchange. Before an IPO, the company will be considered private; afterward, it becomes a publicly listed company.

> The phrase "company goes public on Nasdaq/NYSE/LSE" is more commonly used and maybe more commonly understood. An IPO was initially built to help companies raise a significant amount of capital to scale a business. With the rise of larger pools of private capital, where VC funds and PE funds can easily fund $1B+ rounds, IPOs became more of an exit tool to shareholders and early investors rather than the source of large growth capital. Nevertheless, IPOs are an essential part of the capital circle and provide the opportunity to exit with large gains to shareholders and, with this, introduce new investors to the market. An IPO is also a great way to raise capital from public investors while giving access to high-growth (tech) companies to a larger investor base. During the IPO process, a company's structure will be changed from a private limited company to a public limited company. This, along with information disclosure and expectations on publicly listed companies, sets new standards for companies that have been thus far privately run and funded. It requires strong maturity from companies to go for the IPO.
>
> **Kaidi Ruusalepp**, founder and CEO, Funderbeam

L

Lead investor

The first investor to discover a round, a lead investor typically invests more than other investors. They have greater involvement and take on bigger responsibilities.

Lean startup

This is a methodology developed by Eric Ries that many founders, entrepreneurs and companies use to build out their ideas and businesses by using continuous improvement and innovation. This often involves heavy engagement with and feedback from their customers or users as they build and iterate on their products. The lean startup methodology emphasizes the creation of an MVP, which is a very early, feature-light version of a product that can be shared with alpha and beta testers. The concept is expounded upon at length in the book of the same name.

> The Lean Startup *is an iconic book that outlines how entrepreneurs use continuous innovation to create successful businesses. It has been widely adopted by many in the startup ecosystem, and large*

corporate innovators have recently been treating it as a framework for entrepreneurial endeavors within the enterprise. While the lean startup model is rooted in the concept of launching to learn, corporate innovation teams have over-indexed on the pre-MVP experimentation and consumer validation aspect of the framework and failed to launch. The CFO of a Fortune 50 company recently described this as "experimentation and validation hell".

A corporate innovation team we worked with were essentially stuck in a loop of validating an endless list of leap-of-faith assumptions. A year of validation had passed by before their internal investors asked, "Where is the MVP?" The team answered by outlining the long list of experiments but failed to show an actual MVP that could be iterated on to find product/market fit. Looking back, the team had gathered enough evidence to support the request for MVP build and launch funding (i.e., the venture pitch) nearly a year beforehand. The lesson learned here is that the lean startup entrepreneur always has an eye towards going to market. The market always wins, and the sooner you begin incubating in the market, the sooner you'll be able to tell if you're on the path to success.

Andrew Backs, *founder and chief innovation strategist, Pilot44*

Ledger

The public record of transactions on a blockchain. Ledgers are distributed across numerous computers and can be managed by many people, enabling the blockchain to achieve true decentralization.

Leveraged buyout

Also known as an LBO, this is when a company is acquired (often when a buyer lacks the necessary cash), and a high proportion of the money put into the acquisition is borrowed against the company's assets or cash flow.

Limited partner

An investor in a VC or other fund. Most VC funds raise their capital from limited partners (LPs), including founders, operators, high-net-worth individuals, pension funds, corporations, funds of funds and many others. The term can also be used to refer to a part-owner of a company whose individual liability for the company's debts cannot exceed the amount they've invested in the company itself.

Liquidation

The process of dissolving a company by selling off all of its assets.

Liquidation preference

A clause or term in investment documents and term sheets that relates to the way in which cash or returns are distributed. In many angel and early-stage rounds, investors receive ordinary shares in the company. Later-stage investors often ask for a 1x liquidation preference, which means that they get their exact initial capital back before any cash is distributed to other investors and shareholders. A 2x liquidation preference would mean any investor with this clause in their investment agreement would get twice their investment back before any capital distributions to other shareholders.

LTV

Shorthand for lifetime value. Usually used to refer to your customers, the LTV is the average amount of revenue you'll generate from someone over their lifetime as a paying customer of your business.

LTV/CAC ratio

An equation used to measure the lifetime value of a customer divided by the customer acquisition cost of acquiring that user. A CAC of more than three is considered good. Anything less would not be considered positively once you factor in the non-CAC costs of running a business.

M

Marketplace

A business that facilitates transactions between users. Generally, we think of marketplaces as being two-sided – demand and supply. For example, Pesky Fish is a UK marketplace where the demand side (consumers and hospitality businesses) can buy directly from the supply side (fishermen and port operators). Some on-demand platforms such as Uber Eats, Postmates and others can be viewed as three-sided, with customers, couriers and suppliers all forming part of the value chain.

MAU

An acronym for monthly active users. This is a KPI used to count the number of unique users that visit a site or use an app within a month.

Mentor

An experienced professional who informally helps to guide a less experienced individual or startup in building their venture.

> *By definition, a mentor is an experienced and trusted advisor. In theory, all three elements – experience, trust, advice – contribute to a well-rounded mentor, but there are additional factors to consider. A well-suited mentor will often be referred through a known and trusted network, have experience from a relevant industry and will value your time, be reliable and communicate effectively. A mentor will challenge you, encourage you and work with you to deliver the best results, often both personally and professionally. At Level39, we find that mentors are also fantastic navigators across industries and organizations, offering introductions to their network where appropriate.*
>
> *A mentee should be open to learning from a mentor's past mistakes and failures, positively shaping their business journey. When suitably paired, mentee and mentor relationships can be most rewarding. Startups are the creative innovators of tomorrow, but direction and lessons learnt are always needed along the way.*
>
> **Amy French**, *director, Level39*

Metaverse

A term that was first coined by Neal Stephenson in his sci-fi classic *Snow Crash*. In the book, the metaverse is a virtual world accessed via virtual reality (VR) headsets. The more modern definition maintains that but also adds in the concept of augmented (AR) and mixed reality. Proponents of the metaverse see a future in which the internet evolves into a 3D world accessible via VR headsets, AR goggles and other devices that allow users to access a fully virtual world or a mixed-reality view of the real world. Games such as *Second Life* were early examples of metaverse concepts, but perhaps the most popular depiction came in the book and movie *Ready Player One*.

Mezzanine financing

A form of business financing in which the company that's borrowing pays a higher rate of interest than on other loans. However, they have longer to pay back the debt, which may also be converted into shares in the company.

MVP

Shorthand for minimum viable product. This is a new product that's developed with core features only, in order to measure initial response and collect insights to validate the idea and provide input for future product development.

> In its purest sense, MVP is an idea for a product or service that has been developed into a working solution. Understandably, reaching the MVP stage is an exciting time for the entrepreneur, and essential when seeking new investment, as it's the clearest signal that all the hard work has translated into something tangible. Nevertheless, as someone who has devoted many years to getting brands and agencies to adopt new tech, rarely have I seen a product hit MVP and also be a minimal viable business. Inventing something that appears to deliver on a problem set by the founder must always be put into the perspective of the end buyer of the product.
>
> I'd caution that the investor community threshold for continuing a conversation with an entrepreneur is much lower than for potential clients. Investors can and do get taken in by how "game-changing" and "disruptive" the solution is, the back stories of the founders and exponential growth revenue projections. People diverting funds from elsewhere to purchase your product are not. They want to know that it solves a real, not perceived, challenge for their business. Therefore, the supply-side evidence of an MVP must be accompanied by strong demand-

side proof before founders can honestly say they have a viable business. So, entrepreneurs, when you talk about your MVP to investors and future clients, remember that they're different audiences. For end customers, MVP means evidence of application, proof that your product or service makes a difference (i.e., real-world case histories), a realistic and relatable pricing model and the confidence that your company has the wherewithal to sustain the inevitable test-and-learn problems. Simply put, the same amount of energy the founders have put into developing a "working" product must be matched by a thorough understanding of who and why people will want to buy it.

Jim Kite, *founder, Tech Pilot Ltd; former global head, NextTechNow; head of global partnerships, Publicis Media*

N

NDA

Stands for nondisclosure agreement. This is a legal contract that sets out an agreement regarding the sharing of information or ideas in confidence. For example, if a startup is considering a partnership with a larger corporate entity, they may use an NDA so that the startup can share details of their technology, and the corporation can share details of theirs, without fear of either side copying or disclosing any details that may be detrimental to the interests of one or both parties.

Network effects

These occur when the value of a product or service increases as a result of a higher number of users or participants. For example, owning a telephone has no value unless other people also own telephones. Likewise, marketplace platforms such as Etsy and others require network effects to ensure a balance between buyers and sellers.

NFT games

In NFT games, players can swap or trade the in-game NFTs with other players to earn profits. All rules and conditions within NFT games exist within smart contracts.

Non-fungible token

A token that can be used to demonstrate ownership of unique digital items (e.g., digital art, music, blogs, tickets). A non-fungible token (NFT) can only have one official owner at a time and is usually secured by the Ethereum blockchain.

Oversubscription

When companies set out to raise a round of funding, they typically tell investors a specific amount that they're raising. In many cases, they end up receiving more offers of capital than they originally planned for. In these cases, investors think of the round as oversubscribed, and this creates an opportunity for a founder of a company to negotiate the valuation upward.

P2P

Also known as peer-to-peer, this is a decentralized platform where two individuals can transact directly with each other without the involvement of a third-party intermediary. Some of the most famous examples of P2P businesses include Skype and Napster, as well as more recent examples such as FundingCircle.

Paas

An acronym for platform as a service. This is a category of cloud computing where developers are provided with an on-demand environment with the tools, infrastructure and operating systems for software development over the internet. SAP's Cloud product and Heroku are both examples of PaaS businesses.

Pay to play

Also known as pay to earn, this requires that an investor continues to contribute to financing in order to avoid a penalty for discontinuing finance. It's often a conversion of preferred stock into common stock, which provides a strong incentive for investors to participate in future financings.

Pitch

An opportunity for a startup to present their idea to potential investors, accelerators and entrepreneurs.

The pitch is arguably the most important presentation a startup will have to deliver. A good pitch can lead to many positive outcomes, not least new business and investment opportunities, which are essential ingredients for a successful startup company. In contrast, a bad pitch can leave a company treading water, never quite moving forward and eventually running out of opportunities and money. I've witnessed hundreds of startup pitches and facilitated numerous meetings where a startup is only a pitch away from winning lucrative paid work with a large corporate client. In the vast majority of cases, the best pitch wins the deal, but it isn't always the best tech for the job. I've given up predicting which company from those pitching will come out as the winner. There are too many variables in place. However, I can guarantee that if you follow some simple housekeeping rules, you can greatly improve your chances of succeeding.

The rules are simple: rehearse your presentation thoroughly; arrive early; keep to the time requirements; and always, always, leave time for questions. The discussion time after the pitch is just as important as the pitch itself. These rules are simple but often overlooked. In my experience, one of the biggest reasons why a startup that technically should've won the pitch loses is over-presenting (talking too much) and not leaving enough time for questions afterwards. Losing a pitch because your tech isn't right is one thing; losing it when your tech is perfect but you didn't allow for questions to reconfirm that fact, is criminal. Unfortunately, this scenario is not uncommon, and many startups are left confused as to why an opportunity that is perfect for their offering has (again) not resulted in any new business.

Ken Valledy, *partner/co-founder, Progressive*

Pivot

This is when a company shifts to an alternate business strategy, sometimes completely changing direction, and sometimes to address a specific area. This can be due to customer preference, industry changes or an initial strategy that didn't work.

The original idea behind SoPost was to create a dynamic postal address linked to your social IDs, so that your address became not where you lived but where you wanted your post to be sent. The project dates back to 2009, was the main reason I dropped out of university and was pretty much the sole focus of my life for four years. When I launched SoPost, my main objective was to see whether I'd quit uni for the right reason, and if the idea had legs. I quickly ticked that box, as the concept was validated by every stakeholder I needed. The only problem was that I couldn't figure out how to get to the scale I wanted without millions of dollars of VC funding (which I didn't have).

> At the time of launch, we powered a social gifting marketing campaign for Noel Gallagher's High Flying Birds, which was seen by someone quite high up at Avon Cosmetics. She got in touch and asked if we could adapt what we'd built for her, as she wanted her customers to be able to send a product to a friend, for free. When I visited, I was met by an incredibly successful woman who was really excited and told me that she'd be our first customer (and pay us) if we could do this for her. I had no idea what she was seeing but trusted that she was seeing something that I couldn't. Not knowing how to execute the original vision, I chose the path of least resistance and pivoted. It was only months later that I worked out what was so valuable about what Avon had asked for. That pivot changed the course of my business and was one of the best decisions I ever made.
>
> **Jonathan Grubin**, *founder and CEO, SoPost*

Play to earn

This means that players can earn rewards and even money in the online games that they play. The play-to-earn movement is a rapidly emerging phenomenon in the world of gaming, where players of NFT games can swap or trade in-game NFTs with other players to earn profits.

POC

Stands for proof of concept. The term is generally used when B2B businesses begin to test their product and work with larger corporate or enterprise partners. A proof of concept at this stage is a testing phase where the startup can do a small test to determine the feasibility of a wider partnership or business relationship.

> If your business relies on landing large customers, then step one is usually to get them to try the product. In most situations, depending on the size of the customer, the first step is usually to do a POC. The idea is to make sure that the customer gets to see value. We had to do this multiple times in the initial days, and still do. The hardest part is to make sure that you demonstrate real value without giving away the store!
>
> A POC should ideally be scope limited and budgeted, with clear metrics. You're not doing this as a freebie. Ideally you want the customer to agree about what success looks like as well as the next steps. The reason for this is to make sure that customers are not merely kicking the tires but are actually interested in buying the product! A great POC can immediately launch you into the right conversations. It's a phenomenal tool that we try to use as often as we can. In fact, we came up with an alternative approach by creating a demo site where the client can try our data product and the user experience for themselves and see a sample of the data instantly, with zero friction. We also created an

> analytics demo where the clients can explore the types of insights they can access with our services. The demos got rid of the need for a free POC, which was great. The POCs we do now are simply small-scale, paid pilots so we know that there's skin in the game on the client's side too.
>
> **Shruti Malani Krishnan**, *founder and COO, PY Insights (Powr of You)*

Preferred stock

Preferred stockholders have priority over a company's income and returns, so any dividends or proceeds from an exit are paid out before common stockholders receive their shares. Many investors will ask for preferred stock in their investment agreements at a post-seed stage, and convertible notes will frequently convert into preferred stock.

Pre- and post-money valuation

When a company raises capital, investors can use a pre- or post-money valuation of the company to denote the valuation of that business. A pre-money valuation is the valuation of the company before the value of the investment capital is added in. Post-money valuations include that investment capital value. For example, a post-money valuation of £5M on a £1M raise means the company had a £4M pre-money valuation.

Pre-seed funding

The earliest stage of funding for a new company looking to get started, usually sourced from angels, family and friends (where applicable) and generally excluding any involvement from institutional investors, although there are an increasing number of micro-funds that are catering to pre-seed rounds.

Private equity

Often abbreviated to PE, this refers to investment funds, generally organized as limited partnerships, which buy and restructure companies. A private equity manager typically uses the money of its member investors to fund its acquisitions. Some examples of fund investors are hedge funds, pension funds and high-income individuals. PE funds usually operate at a later stage of the life cycle of a business, where the company has already raised multiple rounds of capital or achieved substantial profitability.

Priced round

A funding round undertaken by a company where the price per share and valuation (or overall price of the company) is defined. This differs from convertible note rounds, where the valuation is formalized in a subsequent funding round.

Product/market fit

Product/market fit refers to a stage in a company's development where the product they have developed fits a clear need in the market. This is generally the stage where the company starts to scale more rapidly, as reaching product/market fit implies that the product now solves a sufficiently large pain point so customers and/or users will be far more likely to download, engage with or purchase the product.

> You have product/market fit (PMF) if 40+ percent of your users would be "very disappointed" if your service shut down tomorrow. Sean Ellis, who led growth at companies like Dropbox and LogMeIn, arrived at this insight after years of trying to define what PMF looked like. You can read more about Sean's "Product Market Fit Test" at **https://blog.growthhackers.com/using-product-market-fit-to-drive-sustainable-growth-58e9124ee8db**, along with an example of how Superhuman adapted it to filter by cohort when determining PMF.
>
> Sean's PMF test has become widely accepted by the startup and investor community as a great way to measure PMF. Another great way is to look for the "Despite Moments". Alex Weidauer, who is the founder and CEO of Rasa.ai (raised $14M in Series A from Accel) and a Techstars Berlin alumnus, first introduced me to his "Despite Moments" idea a few years back when he was mentoring at Techstars.
>
> Alex knew that he and Alan Nichol (his co-

*founder) were on the right path with Rasa when he
noticed that "despite" not having a signup page,
people would seek out their emails and contact
them directly for early access. He noticed more and
more "Despite Moments" where early adopters
encountered friction or other barriers yet still
persevered "despite" the product not offering them
an easy solution. Alex described these "Despite
Moments" as magical early signals that they were on
the right track.*

*They are now what I look for as a founder and
an early-stage investor. Other examples of "Despite
Moments" might be seeing…*

- *users hounding you for early access to a closed
beta*
- *users asking you how they can pay you when you
have no payment pages*
- *users start hacking your product for other use
cases that you don't support (e.g., hashtags in
Twitter)*
- *users spend a lot of time trying to get around a
bug and sending you detailed bug reports*
- *users being happy to attend long onboarding
calls or fill out detailed questionnaires*
- *users complaining about your product but they
keep using it*
- *users spend time exporting and transforming
their data into your format so that they can import
it and play with your product.*

*No founder wants to have "Despite Moments"
(i.e., friction or gaps in their product) but don't forget
'The Alex Weidauer Test' when it happens. Embrace*

these moments for what they are: early signals that you might be on the right path to PMF!

If you have any other examples of "Despite Moments" then I'd love to hear them. You can ping me on Twitter via @ConnorPM

Connor Murphy, *founder, Bridge*

Proprietary

A term used to describe something that belongs to a startup, business or individual. Many machine-learning and AI companies have proprietary algorithms that they use to operate their business. This and other types of proprietary IP are highly valued by investors. Investors also frequently talk about proprietary deal flow, meaning unique access to certain deals.

Pro-rata rights

These are rights given to investors in a company to invest in future rounds of funding so that they can maintain their level of shareholding. It's a right rather than an obligation to invest. Many investors waive their pro rata. Others request super pro rata, where they are given the right to invest more and increase the size of their shareholding in subsequent rounds. However, this is far less common.

Public and private keys

These are the working parts of public key cryptography. Together, they encrypt and decrypt data that exists in a network. The public key can be shared widely, while the private key should only be known by the owner. For example, public keys are like bank account numbers. They can be freely shared with everyone, and anyone can potentially send transactions to them. A private key is like a PIN number, which, together with its corresponding public key information, grants you access to the actual funds in the account.

RAWI

An acronym meaning ready, able, willing, impelled. This is a test that some founders use to decide whether or not they should start a business or expand their business into a new area. The premise is that you need to be ready, able, willing and impelled before you can make the right judgment about what to do.

Reality distortion field

This concept comes from an episode of *Star Trek*, and is commonly used in the tech sector to describe the way in which Steve Jobs was able to convince others to achieve goals and complete tasks that were considered (by people other than Steve Jobs) to be impossible. More recently, it has been used to describe the way in which WeWork's Adam Neumann and Elizabeth Holmes of Theranos were able to pull the wool over the eyes of investors, journalists and stakeholders alike. The most famous example of this came in an interview that Forbes writer Alex Konrad gave for Hulu's documentary *WeWork: Or the Making and Breaking of a $47 Billion Unicorn*. In it, he described how Neumann mixed up cappuccino and latte, leading to team members simply switching the meaning of each word. According to Konrad: "It stood out to me as a strange, gratuitous reality-distortion moment around Adam because he was ordering lattes but wanted cappuccinos. And rather than try to explain to him that he's wrong, they're just going to change the meaning of that word."

Recapitalization

Also known as a recap, this is where a company resets or cleans up its cap table. In this instance, previous investors are heavily or fully diluted to give the founders or new investors a larger share of the equity in the company.

Reverse vesting

This is where a startup employee earns the majority of their options towards the end of their vesting period. In a regular vesting schedule, employees vest over three to four years, with a one-year cliff, which means that they get the right to buy 25 percent of their options at the end of the first year, with the remainder of their options vesting over the following 36 months. In the case of reverse vesting, employees vest smaller amounts in the first period of their employment, with a larger amount (equivalent to the cliff) vesting at the end of a three- to four-year period.

Roadmap

A long-term strategic document that details where your company or product is going, and the necessary major steps required to get there. A roadmap can also be a valuable communication tool for investors, as it helps to articulate strategic thinking behind the goal and the plan for getting there.

> Having a roadmap is a fundamental requirement for any startup or entrepreneur. A roadmap should be a high-level explanation about the future direction of the organization and the development plans that ultimately ladder up to that business achieving its strategic goals. Potential investors will always be looking to understand the long-term plan to gauge the potential return on investment, while corporations assessing whether there's a valid partnership opportunity will want to understand if there will be sustained mutual benefits.
>
> When working for a pet insurance provider, I once assessed a partnership opportunity with a pet-tracking startup. My initial assessment of the technology revealed that their device wasn't providing the clinical-grade data that would make them a valuable partner for me in the short term. They did, however, showcase an impressive roadmap that set out their company vision. It told the story of how their ambition wasn't just to be a pet-tech business focused on the scaling of a single device, but how they wanted to build a whole ecosystem of solutions in the pet health space and eventually own

the category. Seeing that development roadmap help me to understand their vision and strategic direction. Later that year, we cofunded a research project, with the results benefiting both parties. Suffice to say that project wouldn't have gone ahead had that startup not communicated their roadmap and shown how we could learn together.

Jim Edwards, *digital innovation lead EMEA, Kimberly-Clark*

ROFR

Stands for right of first refusal. This allows an individual or business to conduct a business transaction before anyone else – for startups, ROFR offers remaining shareholders the right to purchase shares first, if any other shareholder chooses to sell them before others can do so.

ROI

Stands for return on investment. This is the ratio between net income and an investment, and is habitually used as a sign of the efficiency or impact of investing capital.

Round

Also known as a fundraising round, this is what startups and investors call a qualified financing event, where one or more investors participate at the same time. For example, a startup may do a SEIS round of £150,000 from multiple investors. Once that money is wired and the legal documents associated with the round are signed, that round is deemed to be closed. The next time the company raises money, that triggers another round of funding. Many startups go through multiple rounds of funding: pre-seed, seed, A/B/C/D, bridge rounds, debt rounds and more.

Runway

The amount of time a business can continue operating before it runs out of cash. This is generally a function of how much money a business has in its bank account and its monthly burn rate.

S

SaaS

An acronym for software as a service. This is cloud-based software that is owned, delivered and managed remotely by one or more providers, allowing users to subscribe to applications on a pay-as-you-go basis.

SAFE

Stands for simple agreement for future equity. It's similar to a convertible note in that it's an investment agreement between an investor and a startup. The key difference is that a convertible note is a form of loan that attracts interest and has a maturity date. A SAFE does not.

Scaleup

A stage in a company's growth cycle where it has achieved product/market fit and is scaling rapidly. The term is used to describe companies that, at a minimum, have raised at least a Series A, or companies that have more than £1M or $1M in annual revenue. These businesses are generally seeing substantial growth in their user numbers, revenue, team sizes and more.

SEC

Stands for the Securities and Exchange Commission. This is a US government agency that exists to protect investors, support the fair operation of public and private markets, and facilitate capital formation. Their remit covers everything from insider trading to crowdfunding, and from public markets to startups.

Secondary selling

Where a company, individual or fund sells some or all of their ownership stake to another private investor prior to the company being publicly traded. Secondary sales usually happen in conjunction with funding rounds, allowing founders and early employees to sell some of their shareholding and get some liquidity.

> *The secondary market is where investors buy and sell securities they already own. A secondary transaction is when a new investor buys shares from an existing investor or investors. Secondary transactions or opportunities to sell the existing shares in startup companies mainly occur with new funding rounds. The new investor invests in new shares and buys some shares from the existing shareholder to secure a larger stake in the company. The price is often the same as in the funding round, or slightly discounted. Recently, many secondary funds have been established that buy shares without new funding. The*

funds either find parties interested in selling their shares or are one counterparty in funding rounds but aim for the secondary shares only.

Due to the complexity of selling secondary shares, including tax structures, international law and other restrictions on the sale of shares, many marketplace businesses have started up to help solve these problems and make the process easier for all stakeholders. Some marketplaces provide matching between the seller and the buyer (e.g., ForgeGlobal), some build employee share trading (CartaX) and some run more complex trading pools (Funderbeam). In whichever form, a secondary share transaction is a great opportunity for founders, employees and early shareholders to get some liquidity (cash) before an official exit (merger, acquisition or IPO).

Kaidi Ruusalepp, *founder and CEO, Funderbeam*

Seed round

A funding round that usually involves larger institutional investors. As of 2021, seed rounds in Europe are typically between £1M and £3M, with seed rounds in the US being between $1M and $5M. Seed rounds are generally also the first round in which an investor will require a board seat. Where pre-seed rounds are designed to help companies get the first version of their product to market, a seed round is about getting to product/market fit and preparing for scale.

SEIS

Stands for Seed Enterprise Investment Scheme. This was launched in the UK to encourage investors to finance startups by providing tax breaks for backing projects that may otherwise have been viewed as too risky.

> This UK government tax initiative, together with its EIS big brother, fuels the early-stage UK startup scene. UK angel investors are able to claim a 50 percent tax deduction (SEIS) or 30 percent deduction (EIS) from that year's taxable income (lesser-known fact: they can also backdate the deduction to the previous tax year). If they keep their shares for three years, they pay no capital gains tax on a sale. And, if the company goes out of business, they can write off their investment. We estimate that 80 percent of early stage (sub-£500K rounds) is SEIS/EIS investment. Frankly, it's a complete mystery why every other country hasn't copied the UK scheme (Ireland and Australia, among others, have had a go, but their schemes are garbage, and they are little used).
>
> The SEIS and EIS schemes have some seemingly odd rules, which on closer inspection are cleverly designed to close loopholes in previous HMRC investment schemes. For example, companies that are in oil or gas exploration or electricity generation can't offer SEIS/EIS tax breaks, likely due to the previous VCT investment scheme being exploited by funds setting up special-purpose vehicle energy companies and taking the tax benefits.

> *Some say that SEIS/EIS distorts the UK startup ecosystem ("Do you offer SEIS/EIS? Great, I'm in! Remind me again, what do you do?") and disadvantages companies that don't qualify (notably fintech/banking/leasing/energy). Founders of those companies definitely need to work harder to find investors, but that's minor compared to the huge amount of founder-friendly angel investor money available, which has produced an early-stage UK startup scene that's perhaps the most vibrant anywhere in the world.*

Anthony Rose, *founder and CEO, SeedLegals*

Series

Funding rounds are generally called Series X rounds: Series Seed-funding, Series A/B/C, and so on.

Series A

This is a round of funding of between $5M and $30M. Typically led by institutional investors or VC funds, a Series A is the first stage of growth funding that companies will receive. This is often the round where companies will start to spend larger amounts of money on marketing as they grow and scale.

Series B/C/D

These and subsequent rounds are generally referred to as growth capital, where the capital is used by the company to increase their marketing spend, expand into new markets, acquire other businesses, expand their team and more. For the most part, these companies are already moving towards or are beyond profitability, and are preparing for an exit or IPO as the series moves through the alphabet.

Series C

A funding round that occurs when a company is well established and at the last stage of the growth cycle. This can be due to interest in scaling and expanding success or to address short-term challenges.

Series D

This funding is part of a company's growth capital. Larger venture capital and private equity funds usually participate in a Series D round. Funds generated are used to fuel growth, expansion, acquisitions and preparation for an exit or IPO.

Sidecar fund

See annex fund.

Smart contract

Computer code that automatically executes all or parts of an agreement and is stored on a blockchain-based platform. Unlike traditional contracts, smart contracts don't require the support of third parties or intermediaries.

SME

Shorthand for small- or medium-sized enterprise or business. While many startups would be included in this category, SMEs don't always fall under the high-growth definition of a startup. Most SMEs do not have VC funding.

Smoke testing

A software testing process that determines whether or not a deployed software build is stable. It consists of a minimal set of tests run on each build to test software functionalities. Smoke testing is also known as build verification testing or confidence testing.

Social web

Includes web-based services that enable community-based input and output, such as social networking websites Facebook and Twitter (See: Web 2.0).

Split testing

See: A/B testing.

Stage

Shorthand for the phase of development that a startup has reached. Pre-seed companies are usually at the idea/prototype stage, conducting customer discovery, initial pilots and tests, and iterating their idea. A later-stage company – Series A/B/C onwards – has generally reached product/market fit and is now rapidly scaling its business.

Startup

A new company or recently created business looking for a business model that is repeatable and scalable.

Static web

A collective term for websites that are delivered to every web browser and remain the same for every user (See: Web 1.0).

Stock options

Also known as options, these are a benefit frequently given to early-stage startup employees or advisors, although some large companies such as Amazon, Facebook and others will give equivalent grants in the form of RSUs (restricted stock units). An option gives the grantee the right to purchase those shares at a pre-agreed (typically low) price at some point in the future. Stock options are normally expressed in percentage terms or in terms of the number of shares being offered to an employee. Most stock options vest over a one- to four-year period, meaning that an employee earns the right to all of the stock options they've been offered over that period of time. Stock options are usually subject to a cliff (meaning that up to a year passes before you start vesting), have a strike price (the price per share that has been pre-agreed) and an exercise period (meaning that you have a limited time period to buy the stock at the agreed price after you leave a company). Option owners can have a substantial financial outcome in the event of working at a successful company where the share price increases substantially, while the option holder still has the right to buy shares at a far lower price and then sell them for a substantial profit. For example, early team members become millionaires (and in some cases, billionaires) when they sell their early options in the company after its IPO.

Sweat equity

When you give shares in your company to early employees or contractors in place of cash. It's a common practice in startups that haven't yet raised funds. If you take a chance with a startup, your shares might become lucrative when the company sells.

> On paper, sweat equity is attractive to an early-stage business where funding is tight but their plans need to be accelerated. If a required service can be provided for equity rather than paid for from company funds, then surely it's a no-brainer?
>
> The pitfall is that whoever is providing the service is typically doing so in their downtime, which means it isn't prioritized in the same way as paid work. Corners can be cut and timeframes not met because the service provider needs to earn a living or generate a profit. If possible, I'd suggest steering clear of sweat equity. Focus on fundraising and perhaps consider raising at a reduced valuation to generate enough funds to allow you to reach the next significant milestone. If that's not achievable, then use sweat equity as a fallback. If it becomes necessary, stay close to the sweat equity provider. Scrutinize their work early on and continue to scrutinize it. If you see a lack of quality, or deadlines start to be missed, then you should be concerned. Try to resolve any challenges early on and make sure you have some form of get-out agreement regarding quality and timings to allow you to walk away if you need to.
>
> **Howard Simms**, co-founder and director, Apadmi

Switching costs

The difficulty or costs (psychological, financial, effort- and time-based) that are incurred by switching from one product or service to another.

T

TAM

An acronym for total addressable market. This is usually used to describe the revenue opportunity obtainable for a product or service - or the total demand that exists in a market for it.

( )tech

There are many subsectors of the technology industry. There are various terms which are portmanteaus of the word "tech" preceded by the sector that company is working in or targeting. The best known of these is fintech. Companies in that sector include businesses such as Transferwise, Revolut, Cuvva, Monzo and many others, all companies that are innovating in, partnering with or disrupting established companies in the finance sector. There are several other examples, including cleantech (companies that are working towards a cleaner environment and substantial energy savings), adtech (advertising), edtech (education), and insurtech (insurance), to name but a few.

Term sheet

A document outlining the terms and conditions of a potential business agreement, setting out the basis for future negotiations between the seller and the buyer. It's usually the first documented evidence of a possible investment or acquisition and can be binding or nonbinding.

Tough tech venture

Technology that's considered to be transformative. A tough tech venture often requires more time to get off the ground, as well as increased rounds of development and experimentation.

Tranches

Tranches refer to when an investor commits to financing but does not offer all the money to a business all at once. Each portion, or tranche, is released only when the company hits agreed-upon targets.

UHNWI

Shorthand for ultra-high-net-worth individual. To be a UHNWI, you need to have at least $30M worth of net investable assets in your name. However, this is only a guide, as there's no standard legal threshold. As the name would suggest, UHNWIs are the wealthiest people in the world.

Unicorn

A privately held startup company valued at more than $1B.

Unit economics

A way of measuring the profitability (or potential profitability) of a company. The unit economics are calculated by looking at the revenue and costs associated with your business. For example, in a SaaS business, each customer could be defined as a unit, so the calculation of the value of each unit is the LTV of that customer minus their CAC. This is also referred to as contribution margin.

Up round

A round of financing in which the company's worth has gone up since its previous valuation.

Upstream integration

When a company begins to control more of the component parts of their business. For example, a direct-to-consumer business might buy their own manufacturing equipment rather than outsourcing, or a SaaS company might build their own internal tools rather than using third-party ones.

V

Validated learning

This allows you to quantify and (dis)prove a hypothesis. If you conduct 50 user interviews about a new feature and 80 percent of people say they wouldn't pay for it, that can be seen as a validated learning. Likewise, you can use split tests on your website to get validated learning about conversion rates and more.

Valuation

A phrase used to describe the current, actual or theoretical worth of a company. Many methods are used to value a company. In public markets, multiple data points can be used to determine the valuation (or market cap) of a company. This is a far more difficult thing to determine in pre-seed and seed-stage companies, where the valuation is frequently determined by the momentum of a company and the degree of excitement or hype that surrounds that business.

VC

Short for venture capital. This is an asset class that is focused on investing in earlier-stage, illiquid assets such as startups. Venture capital is generally a higher-risk investment, as there's a substantial failure rate with early-stage businesses compared to publicly traded or other liquid assets. Venture capital is typically deployed via funds that pool capital from LPs and then have their team and partners invest in the companies on their behalf. VC funds can be generalist or sector/stage/geography-specific.

VCT

Stands for venture capital trust. This refers to an investment vehicle that operates in the United Kingdom. The VCT is a closed-end fund that was created by the UK government in the 1990s to help drive direct investment into local private businesses. These funds are tax efficient and allow individual investors to access venture capital investments via capital markets. VCTs seek out potential venture capital investments in small, unlisted firms that are in their early stages to generate higher-than-average, risk-adjusted returns. VCTs are commonly listed on the London Stock Exchange (LSE).

Venture debt

A type of financing provided to startups by specialist lenders and banks. It's generally raised alongside an equity funding round and is used to cover working capital or capital expenditure for equipment, etc. The main difference between venture lending and more traditional bank loans is that venture debt providers typically work with companies that are not cash-flow positive or are at an earlier stage. Venture debt providers also take warrants to invest in companies and can end up owning substantial stakes if repayments are not kept up.

Vertical

Used to describe a group of companies that focus on a shared niche. Many VC funds, accelerators or CVCs are vertical or sector-specific, with a focus on sectors such as fintech, healthtech, medtech and so on (See: ( )tech).

Vertical integration

When a company extends all operations to ensure that it's in control of the full supply chain, from manufacturing to end sales.

Vesting

A legal term that means to give or earn the right to a present or future payment, stock, asset or benefit. In startup employee agreements, people are paid a combination of salary and stock options. Those options give employees the right to buy equity in the company at an agreed (often discounted) rate. In most cases, those options vest or accrue to the employee over a given period of time, usually three to four years.

Web 1.0

The first stage of the evolution of the internet. In the early days of the World Wide Web, there were only a few content creators. It was a one-to-many model, with the majority of people consuming. For the most part, Web 1.0 sites were static pages with little or no user interaction.

Web 2.0

Also known as the social web, this is the second stage of development of the internet, characterized by the transition from static web pages to dynamic or user-generated content. It heralded the rapid growth of social media and other services, which ran on the basis of gaining access to personal data for advertising purposes.

web3

This is the third evolution of the web, which has blockchain as its backbone, offering a governance layer for trusted transactions. It's built upon the core concepts of decentralization, openness and greater user utility – a decentralized network without the need for third parties.

White label

This type of technology is a ready-made licensed software product developed by one company and then rebranded by another, to appear as its own.

Acknowledgments

I couldn't have completed this book without the help of many people. First and foremost, my wife, Katie, and my daughters, Charlotte and Annabel, for not only giving me the space but also having the patience to help me to get through this process.

Thanks to Matt Nicholls, my business partner at Progressive, for his continued support with this project, and also to Charlotte, our innovation strategist, who provided invaluable support at the start of the project when our definitions needed to be compiled and checked.

Thanks to the hundreds, if not thousands, of startups that I've met and spoken to over the past eight years. Without these conversations, this book would never have been written.

Thanks to Eamonn, for agreeing to meet for a coffee at very short notice, listening to my idea for this book and, without any fuss, agreeing to jump on board. A different response would've killed this idea for good.

Thanks to Paul and James at The Allotment brand design company for their superb front and back cover designs.

And finally, thanks to Sue, Bev, Andrew and Paul at The Right Book Company. Without their help and guidance, this project would never have crossed the line and would have remained a pipe dream.

Ken Valledy

To Mum and Dad - thanks for the Spectrum and all the computers, internet connections, books, magazines and more. Far more than that, thank you for the support and love that allowed me to do the crazy things that led me to this point.

To Rachael - thanks for putting up with my various harebrained schemes and ideas and for tolerating the majority of them. You're pretty neat.

To Ned - by the time you're old enough to read this, these words will probably look like the cave paintings in Lascaux, but this is all for you.

Thanks to my colleagues and the founders I've been lucky enough to invest in and mentor at Techstars, The Fund and now Tera Ventures! I feel as if you're a huge reason why we've written this book, and also a source of inspiration for so many of the definitions.

Thanks to Sue, Bev, Andrew, Paul and everyone at The Right Book Company for helping us make this a reality. Sorry for the occasional moments of stress. Hopefully this is the first of many collaborations.

Finally, and most importantly, thanks to Ken for coming out to the Angel for a coffee and a chat about an idea that turned into this book!

Eamonn Carey

In addition, we would both like to thank everyone who took time out to contribute stories and testimonials: Emma Jones, Jim Edwards, Shameen Prashantham, Raph Crouan, Shruti Malani Krishnan, Daniel Glazer,

Jonathan Grubin, Christina Richardson, Andrew Backs, Amy French, Jim Kite, Howard Simms, Mick Doran, Andrus Oks, Anthony Rose, Monty Munford, Ian Hathaway, Connor Murphy, Kaidi Ruusalepp, Tom Eisenmann, Nicola Burnside, Matthew Fitzpatrick, Jenny Fielding.

CPSIA information can be obtained
at www.ICGtesting.com
Printed in the USA
BVHW050844020223
657603BV00015BA/78